YOGA FOR TODAY

YOGA
FOR
TODAY

by

CLARA SPRING

and

MADELEINE GOSS

HOLT, RINEHART AND WINSTON
NEW YORK   CHICAGO   SAN FRANCISCO

To

BLANCHE DE VRIES

*Pioneer teacher of Yoga
in the West*

Acknowledgment

We wish to express our special appreciation to Dr. Franklyn Thorpe, distinguished physician and surgeon, for his helpful cooperation in presenting the anatomical and physiological aspects of Hatha Yoga from a scientific point of view.

Introduction

It has been said that Dr. Oliver Wendell Holmes when asked near the end of his long life, "What is man?" answered without hesitation, "A series of states of consciousness." Nothing, to my mind, proves the truth of this statement more conclusively than the simple fact that I now find myself introducing a work such as this.

Over twenty-five years ago, shortly after finishing a long and intensive course of medicine, I found my sister enthusiastically practicing and teaching Hatha Yoga. I remember very clearly taking a dim view of what she was doing with her life. Having just had eight long years of concentrated medical science—with all its various "ologies" drilled into me—I was in no mood to listen to anything which sounded so empirical as the theory and practice of Yoga; I felt that it was faddish and cultish. My "state of consciousness" then was the theory and practice of medicine, surgery, and the operating room.

Never in my wildest flight of fancy could I have imagined actually practicing Yoga myself. A few years ago I heard the late John Van Druten say in his address to the Vedanta Society in Hollywood that in looking back at his early background and scholastic training the least likely thing that he could possibly imagine himself ever doing would be addressing an audience on the subject of Yoga.

Realizing today that Yoga is not only unique but is as profound a science as exists for integrating mind, body, and spirit into a harmonious whole, I have to smile when I recall my youthful ignorance and intolerance. As far as the comparative value of what one does with one's life is concerned, whether in preventing illness and maintaining health in others or helping them by medical means to regain their health after they have become ill, perhaps the edge lies a little on the side of helping others hold on to their most precious possession and teaching them its value.

Looking at the world from a broad aspect and at our own society in particular one must admit that it definitely shows signs of inner sickness and decadence—in spite of undeniable progress on the outer or material side. The consensus of the most mature and foresighted minds of today unquestionably bears this out. We ourselves are inwardly confused and in conflict, full of fear and tension. It is we who make society and the world—in fact, we are society and the world—hence the condition in which we find ourselves, with mental disease, alcholism, psychosomatic disorder, crime, delinquency, mental immaturity, and escapism of every kind increasing out of all proportion to the increase in population.

For those who are statistically minded, figures show some arresting facts which should be more generally known and faced. More hospital beds are occupied by mental cases than by all other diseases combined, including cancer, heart, lung, and polio. We have the highest per-capita rate in the world for crime, chronic alcoholism, and automobile accidents; and this rate is rising year by year.

The increasing number of young men and women rejected by our Army and Navy because of physical and mental disqualifications is also significant. True, we have prolonged our life span by some ten or twelve years in the past few decades, but it is also undoubtedly true that about as many in the fifty-five- to sixty-five-year age bracket die from lack of a feeling of further usefulness as they do from degenerative and geriatric diseases. Who wants to exist like a zombi, whose mind and spirit are dead, but whose body lives on?

We do not like to face unpleasant facts. We are only too ready to listen to the apostles of positivism with their programs of wishful thinking, ego inflation, self-hypnosis, and so-called "right thinking," but it is going to take a much more realistic approach to effect any worth-while change in ourselves. We cannot do it by leaning upon tranquilizing pills, relaxing pills, mood-elevating pills, sedative pills, appetite-reducing pills, alcohol, or other crutches which, after all, are only forms of escapism and self-delusion.

Today in medicine, the best minds, even those of highly developed specialists, are beginning to view the human being as an integrated whole whose mind and body are one and cannot be treated separately with any hope of effective therapy. Many friends of mine specializing in different branches of medicine have told me that about fifty per cent of the patients they see are psychosomatic cases. My own experience as a physician and in twenty-five years of practice bears this out.

In the more than ten years I have been practicing Hatha Yoga almost daily for forty minutes upon arising, I feel that I have had the opportunity to give it the acid test from the standpoint of theory and practice as well as from that of anatomy and physiology. During this period I have rarely had a cold and no diseases of any kind. What has been perhaps of even greater value to me in this confused, fear-ridden world is my concomitant sensitive improvement in mental and emotional control and self-knowledge. It has given me a reserve of mental and physical energy and an inner harmony and poise. While saving myself much useless emotional wear and tear during trying and difficult times, the equanimity and imperturbability I have gained has enabled me, through a more patient and sympathetic understanding, to be of infinitely more help to my patients.

While imperturbability and equanimity have always been essential for the survival of the physician, they are of no less importance to the layman. They are as necessary in adversity as in success and prosperity. Imperturbability is almost a physical quality— coolness and presence of mind under all circumstances, calmness amid storm, clearness of judgment in moments of danger. We can develop this quality which will enable us to preserve our individuality and serenity under the rushing stream of other people's personalities, emotions, and hysterias constantly flowing over us. The mental equivalent of imperturbability is equanimity. This enables us to struggle on cheerfully, not just in fair weather, but when the odds seem against us, facing the challenge and conflict of life with our heads up and a smile for the other fellow. In order to have something to give out of physical and mental stability and strength to those near and dear to us, we must devote a certain amount of time to recharging our batteries with energy, to re-creating our bodies and re-collecting our minds in the literal sense of the word.

Although the following chapters cover the subject of Hatha Yoga very thoroughly, I should like to emphasize some of the points which I found helpful as a beginner. Unless and until you make up your mind to practice the exercises slowly, patiently, quietly, gently, persistently—almost as a prayer—there is really no use in beginning at all. There is nothing dramatic, acrobatic, or spectacular about these exercises—they are beautiful and exciting, physically and mentally cleansing and stimulating. There is nothing occult or mysterious about them. They are not intended to be performed as a feat to excite the wonder or envy of friends. The beginner's attitude of mind may not seem important, but I can assure you that it is. The practice of Yoga follows natural laws, older than man himself, which unfortunately most of us have been too slothful or self-indulgent to obey.

The exercises are not intended to develop bunches of muscles like those of a weight lifter or a shot-putter, but they will give you a strong, vital, well-poised body with good muscular tone and reserve strength which is under your command to carry out your will.

What began as a chore I didn't have time for soon became a necessity equal to bathing, care of the teeth, or any of the other cleansing functions of the body. Even today, after ten years, I look forward each morning to the forty minutes of Yoga exercises, followed by a few minutes of meditation and prayer, as the finest hour of the day. My morning starts with an inner feeling of tranquility and even of exhilaration which lasts throughout the day.

Of course, as a beginner, I went through the customary phases of discouragement and impatience. My teacher performed the exercises and postures with such apparent effortlessness, grace, and perfection that I thought it would be impossible for me ever to do them well. The neophyte is apt to lose sight of the years of self-discipline, patience, and effort needed to attain this degree of perfection. These are some of the finest and most valuable achievements of Yoga which are not superficially apparent in the early stages. Some of the exercises I thought I could not master, I now do with ease. Some I do not do as well as I would like, but do them as well as I can. Some that required considerable will, concentration, and persistent effort in the beginning now seem quite simple.

During the years I have been practicing Hatha Yoga, I have lost about four inches around the waist and about fourteen pounds in weight, mostly around the middle. This I attribute mostly to the breathing exercises, for I have never been on a diet of any kind. It is true that I have always enjoyed swimming, riding, and playing tennis with fair regularity, but in addition to my feeling of exuberant health and well-being, it is also mighty fine at my age to be able to undertake pack trips in the High Sierras or practice Hatha Yoga in my hotel room in Mexico City with pleasure and anticipation and without fear of physical exhaustion.

The *Kybalion* (Hermetic) , written about the time of Abraham, some 2500 B.C. says, "When the ear of the disciple is ready, the teacher will appear." Later during the Golden Age of Greece, around 500 B.C., some wise man noted, "Healthy mind, healthy body." Buddha said, "Sloth is man's greatest sin." Still later, Christ preached, "The spirit is willing but the flesh is weak." To our ears these truths may sound obvious. So did most of the truths of the great avatars and sages who tried to teach the world a few simple, clear-cut truths which are as true today as they were in the beginning, for truth is forever what "is" and not what we would like it to be. To live and grow requires effort. This simple fact cannot be escaped nor changed by any form of sophistry, self-deception, wishful thinking, nor magic pills. Hatha Yoga offers a short cut to a healthy life, if the ear of the listener is open. For those who are ready to listen the price of the effort will be repaid many fold.

There is an efficiency which is inspired by love, which is much greater than that motivated by ambition.

There is an achievement and fulfillment in the doing which is greater than the goal.

There is a Self Realization based upon self knowledge which is greater than self improvement.

FRANKLYN THORPE, M.D., F.A.C.S.

Contents

PART III—KEY OUTLINE

Illustrations

Foreword

Many people, hearing of the remarkable results that follow the practice of Yoga, have wanted to know more about this ancient science. Recently a number of popular books have appeared, but these for the greater part stress personal experience rather than practical application, and give only a limited interpretation of the subject.

On the other hand, original texts on Yoga are scarce and hard to find, and they are filled with Sanskrit terms and esoteric symbology that the Western mind finds difficult either to interpret or to apply to practical use.

The present volume, based on long years of study and teaching and founded on authentic sources, has been written in response to a wide demand for a workable text on the physical aspect of Yoga. It presents the basic truths of this time-tested science in simple, streamlined form, together with detailed instructions for the various practices. The text can be read without a Sanskrit dictionary, and the exercises may be put to practical use by following simple directions. This is Yoga adapted to present-day needs: ancient wisdom in modern terms.

In the Orient, Yoga has always been taught by the master-pupil (*Guru-Chela*) method, the student's main requirements being trust in the teacher and belief in the precepts taught. In other words, unquestioning faith.

We of the West, however, are not willing to accept facts blindly. We live in a scientific and rational age, and must prove things to the satisfaction of the intellect. Because of this characteristic we know that, while outer direction is always helpful, the initiative and the ultimate governing factor must lie within ourselves. Our so-called higher self must be the *Guru*, controlling and directing the everyday, material self, or *Chela*.

This does not mean that a teacher is unnecessary. It is quite true that more rapid progress can be made under the direction of a master. But unfortunately there are few sincere and competent teachers to be found in the Western hemisphere, or even in India today for that matter, and we must increasingly depend on the wisdom and direction handed down to us through the written word.

This book presents the physical practices of Yoga in clear, concise style, describing them first in their original form and then including certain adaptations or variations so that everyone, young or old, who is fundamentally sound can make use of the principles involved. For by varying the intensity with which it is performed, Yoga can be practiced when no other kind of exercise is possible. Those who are past fifty will find the work of particular value in helping them to delay the disintegrating forces of old age. Also people who are under par physically can gain great benefit, provided they will use judgment in adapting the work to their individual capacity.*

The exercises have been grouped for convenience under certain general headings. But this listing is only a means of presenting the work and is not intended as the order in which they should be practiced. While the work is entirely authentic, the naming, grouping, and sequence are purely arbitrary, and only classified in this way for practical use.

With all beginners moderation and persistence are of utmost importance. The simpler, easier exercises should be mastered before overenthusiastically attacking the more difficult ones.

Part I deals with the theory, Part II the technique with a full description of each practice. At the end will be found a key outline or summary of the exercises, intended as a chart for daily practice, and referring back to the detailed descriptions and directions for each exercise. A suggested sequence for beginners is also included.

In short, the material is so organized and explained that any intelligent and physically normal man or woman can begin the training and go some distance alone. Actually, books can only point the way. Yoga must be lived in order to be understood. Experience alone will furnish the proof of its validity.

---

* The advisability of a preliminary check-up by a competent physician is important before beginning any new form of exercise.

Part I—*The Theory*

I

Efficient Living

This hill though high I covet to ascend;
The difficulty will not me offend;
For I perceive the way of life lies here.
Come, pluck up, heart; let's neither faint nor fear.
—*Pilgrim's Progress*, John Bunyan

IN ORDER to cope with the speed and pressure of modern life, we must get the most possible out of the equipment and material we have to work with.

There is not enough time in one brief life span to master all knowledge. Today, we have condensed and made available for our immediate benefit, the results of years of research in science and medicine, together with the accumulated wisdom of the ages. Even our reading matter is shortened into digests so that we may be saved time and effort in assimilating new ideas.

In every department of living we have to make use of the short-cut principle. To succeed in any direction we must become "efficiency experts."

Efficient living is only possible where there is enough driving force. Without it nothing worthwhile can be accomplished; even the smallest undertaking becomes an effort. Energy is the creative principle that underlies all success.

3

ENERGY

Energy exists within and all around us. Various outer forms, such as electricity, have been harnessed and made to serve mankind. Latent within ourselves is the greatest energy of all, the universal force that drives the mainspring of all life. By learning how to tap this energy we can become veritable dynamos of power.

While energy is the current that drives the motor, unless it is brought under control and wisely directed it is of no practical use, and may even burn up the motor that produces it. If we wish to be successful in life we must learn to apply energy intelligently.

A strong body, clear mind, and controlled emotions are necessary for any kind of enduring achievement. Too often certain of our faculties have been developed at the expense of others. In concentrating our attention on outer efficiency and worldly success we have sacrificed health, vitality, peace of mind, and joy in living. Our physical equipment has not been equal to the strain we have put upon it.

A way should be found to augment rather than deplete our faculties—physical, mental, and emotional. We must seek a method that will develop energy and at the same time enable us to control and direct the power it produces.

Such a method does exist.

THE WAY

Through a special training based on sound and scientific laws, man can develop extraordinary individual power, bringing to him the fulfillment of his highest potentialities.

This is not a modern discovery. On the contrary, it is a well-known way of life, a centuries-old path, well-trodden and proven by those who have had the enterprise and intelligence to follow it.

Although it is an ancient system, it uses the short-cut principle so necessary in successfully meeting life today. Like all short cuts, however, this path is not a smooth highway where crowds travel and traffic is heavy. It is steep and rugged—not for those who seek the way of least resistance, but far speedier in reaching the ultimate goal.

This path is called Yoga. Those who follow it become efficiency experts in the art of living.

II

What Is Yoga?

If you go where few have gone,
You will find what few have found.
—Gautama Buddha

LITERALLY TRANSLATED, Yoga means "union" or "contact." Our word yoke comes from the same Sanskrit root. Yoga might be called the bridge between the microcosm and the macrocosm, between man's individual soul and universal consciousness. The aim of Yoga is to unite body, mind, and spirit through a system that encompasses all three of these in a psycho-physical method of training.

The origins of Yoga go so far back into antiquity that they have been lost in the passing centuries. Certain sages of India, devoting their lives to a study of man's nature and problems, gradually evolved an organized system of control by means of which he could raise his capacities to their highest level.*

Through the ages this science was jealously guarded, for Yoga gives power, and should never be used for selfish purposes. It was taught only to those who, after long apprenticeship, proved themselves worthy to receive the training.

Because in the past this power has at times been misused, some

* Patanjali was the first to record this method. See: *The Yoga Aphorisms of Patanjali.*

5

people have gained a wrong idea of Yoga. They think of it as a form of cheap magic, fit only for charlatans, or as an ascetic practice followed only by fanatics. But such a distorted picture is far from the real truth. The standards of Yoga are among the highest that man is capable of attaining. The very first requisites of a student (*Chela*), are integrity of character, good will toward all, and a strong moral resolve to learn and to progress.

In the East, definite rules of conduct and inner control are given the student to master. These rules (*Yama-Nyama**), like the Ten Commandments of the Christian religion, the Buddhistic Eight-Fold Path, and Confucius' Laws of Manu, are guides to the highest ethical development. The *Yamas* include harmlessness, truth, honesty, chastity, forgiveness, endurance, compassion, sincerity, frugality, and cleanliness; and the *Nyamas* include discipline, contentment, belief in God, charity, adoration, listening to Truth, modesty, intellect, meditation.

To gain real or lasting benefit from the practice of Yoga, a student must have exceptionally high moral standards.

YOGA—PHILOSOPHY OR RELIGION?

Yoga is not a philosophy, though its practice will lead to a way of life that is philosophical; nor is it a religion. It has no priests nor churches, and it is not confined to any special creed or dogma. There is nothing in the essential principles of this time-honored system that is antagonistic to any religious belief or code of ethics. Where religion is based on faith, a belief that man will ultimately attain a higher state than he is now capable of reaching, Yoga shows a way of proving that faith, demonstrating that the same truth underlies all religions.

For truth in any tongue, in any time or country, remains the same. What is true to us personally is what we can understand, but it has value only if we can use it. An abstract knowing about a subject is not enough. We must live with it and apply it, and thereby prove its truth for ourselves.

In Yoga, realization through practice takes the place of blind faith. Everything here is demonstrable. Results are what count,

---

* *Yama:* death—to bad character qualities. *Nyama:* birth—to good character qualities.

and these may be verified by anyone who with patient and persevering effort is willing to carry through the prescribed work.

There is no easy road to higher powers. We have not yet come to realize our own potentialities. Yoga, by strengthening and disciplining the body and the mind, helps to develop the powers that exist naturally within us.

The training includes every part of man's nature. For Yoga is a way of life that takes into consideration every aspect of a human being.

To suit varying temperaments and capacities, different "paths," or Yogas, have been devised.

THE DIFFERENT YOGAS

Bhakti Yoga, the way of love and devotion, is for those who have religious or emotional natures, such as philanthropists, idealists, artists—all those who devote their lives to a cause.

Karma Yoga brings realization through action. The businessman, householder, or worker in any field, can here find fulfillment.

Jnana Yoga, or the path of the intellect, is suited to scholars, scientists, inventors, and mathematicians. It is the intellectual means to perfection.

Mantra Yoga deals with the science of sound or vibration, both outer—as in speech, music, poetry, drama, spoken prayer—and inner (also known as *Laya Yoga*) —as in religious study and silent prayer.

Raja Yoga, the Path of Kings or Royal Road, is the Yoga of creative imagination and meditation, and is for those who by disciplining their natures have attained nobility of soul.

Hatha Yoga is fulfillment through physical perfection. It is sometimes called the Path of Courage.

The final end of all these paths is union with higher consciousness, and it is possible, through dedicated effort, to reach this goal through any one of the different Yogas. But life is short and there is much to be accomplished, so it is quicker and easier to follow the way best suited to the individual nature and temperament. Nevertheless, an understanding of all the Yogas is important. For example, the *Bhakti* should have some knowledge of *Jnana Yoga* in order to worship intelligently and of *Karma Yoga* so that through discriminative action he may put to use the fruits of his devotion.

Whatever path may be chosen, in the last analysis success is largely dependent on the quality of the instrument through which we are obliged to function. The potentialities of a human being can never be consistently realized until his physical instrument is brought under control. We should first give attention to the body and bring it to a high state of functioning, so that we may be released from its demands and be free to turn our minds to more essential things. Paradoxically, we must remember the body in order to forget it.

A STRONG BODY IS IMPERATIVE

Some people argue that since great things have been accomplished by men with weak or inferior physical equipment it is therefore unnecessary to consider the instrument through which we function. Genius does sometimes demonstrate what can be done with an inefficient vehicle; on the other hand, the average person seldom uses to the utmost the capacities with which he is born, since man is inherently lazy and tends to follow the line of least resistance.

Those with diseased or defective bodies who put forth greater-than-average effort to overcome their condition often compensate for their deficiencies and accomplish more than their less-handicapped fellow men. But who can say how much further these same men might have gone if they had enjoyed perfect health and still applied the same effort?

It is only possible to live to one's fullest capacity when the body is strong and functioning properly. If it is sluggish or diseased one becomes a slave to its insistent aches and pains and cannot direct the mind efficiently, for an unhealthy body creates unhealthy emotional states, and these in turn affect the mind and wear out the body. The ideal is to possess an instrument so finely attuned and so free from inhibiting desires that it becomes one with the goal of the mind. In other words, the practice of Yoga results in a well-integrated personality.

Everyone wants an efficient, well-trained mind, but the fact is overlooked that mind power is really an end product. Just as steam is energy created by raising its basic element, water, to the highest degree of which it is capable, so mental force can be heightened by raising its fundamental, the body, to the ultimate of its capacities.

Our minds and bodies have too often been divorced. Only by joining the two can we secure the great benefits to be gained from a psycho-physical union. This is what Yoga in its basic, or physical, aspect seeks to do.

HATHA YOGA

Hatha comes from two Sanskrit words: *Ha*, meaning the sun or positive principle, and *Tha*, the moon or negative side. These are symbolic of the personal and the universal principles that exist throughout the universe, and are in man's nature as well. Through the union of the negative and the positive, the power of creation can be unlocked. Hatha Yoga is the means by which the body and spirit are joined together, bringing spiritual unfoldment as well as physical perfection.

There are seven steps in the practice of Hatha Yoga. First, the body is purified; second, it is strengthened; third, it is taught outer control; fourth, nerve control; fifth, the body is made light through breathing; sixth, it learns to use its powers objectively through concentration; and seventh, it turns these powers inward, toward spiritual development.

Hatha Yoga specifically teaches control of the body, mind, and emotions. At the same time it builds reserve strength; arrests the tearing-down forces of life and prolongs youth; trains the mind to a steadfast one-pointedness, and brings poise and equanimity to the personality together with increased awareness and a new understanding of life and its laws.

> People have forgotten what the savage instinctively knows: that a perfect body is the supreme instrument of life.
>
> —Havelock Ellis

III

Principles and Training

Whether young or old, sick or lean, one who discards laziness gets success if he practises Yoga. . . .

How can one get success without practice; for by merely reading books on Yoga one can never get success.

—*Hatha Yoga Pradipika*

THERE ARE THREE main principles in the physical training of Yoga. Purification, that is, keeping the system thoroughly clean; control, accomplished through postures and exercises; and breathing, to stimulate the nerve centers.

Our Western physical-culture systems are mainly concerned with outer strength, but this type of exercise often wears down more than it builds up. Everyone, regardless of individual ability, is expected to follow the same drills, and thus a good deal of time and effort are wasted, for no two human beings are exactly alike, nor have they identical capacity.

In Hatha Yoga there is no waste effort. Results are obtained with a minimum of time, space, and activity. Each practice is specific, and brings more than one benefit. For example the "runner's breath" (*Bhastrika*), performed in sitting posture, gives all the

10

advantages of deep breathing obtained in running without the physical depletion caused by violent exertion. Yoga is the most economical yet most intense form of exercise, and the best method ever devised for gaining control of all the bodily functions. It is the short cut to physical perfection.

Some people resist any form of exercise. Even mention of the word creates antagonism, for to them exercise means an unnatural and strenuous throwing around of the body, with sore muscles and general discomfort following.

This is not true of Yoga. Here there is no violent jerking or angular type of movement, but a sustained, even, smooth control that enables the circulation to adapt with a minimum of effort. Since special attention is given to elimination, the fatigue substances—usual by-products of exercise—are carried off instead of remaining in the body to create soreness and fatigue.

HEALTH DEPENDS ON INNER STRENGTH

Outward strength of the body has actually little to do with health. The vital organs such as the heart, liver, kidneys, intestines, etc., are not greatly affected by movements of the arms and legs, and the external muscles play a comparatively small part in maintaining health. Health depends primarily on the condition inside the trunk, between neck and hips.

We in the West are too concerned with outer appearances and effects. Yoga's aim is internal harmony and health, control of the nervous system rather than the development of surface muscles, conservation of energy instead of depletion.

Although the work is almost entirely within the body, the external contour is the first to change. Weight is increased or decreased according to the normal requirements of the individual. Where ordinary routines for reducing often bring a corresponding loss of vitality and a lowered resistance to disease—sometimes with definite injury to health—Yoga practices develop energy as weight is controlled.

From a health angle alone these exercises have such value that most Western physical-culture systems, including the Army "daily dozen," have adopted some of the principles in their routines. Also a number of world-famous beauty courses contain certain exercises based on Yoga.

Most people drift with the tide and grow old before their time. Yoga, by reversing life's processes, offsets nature's destructive forces. All things have two motions: one toward building up: life; and the other toward dissolution: death. In normal health there is a balance between the two; the body builds up as fast as it tears down. But with advancing years the disintegrating forces gain the ascendancy.

To be healthy the body must be used. If unused, various degrees of atrophy, disfunction, and degenerative diseases set in. Yoga is not content with the so-called normal standard of health (which is usually taken from the lowest average) but demands something far beyond. We usually consider ourselves well if we are without pain. There is a state as far above ordinary health as this latter is above disease.

We should not accept with complacency fatigue, headaches, harried nerves, constipation, obesity (with consequent increased susceptibility to disease) or even be satisfied with a condition that at its best is merely pain free. Nor need we fear the disintegration of old age. Old age is purely relative, many are older at forty than others at eighty. It is the quality of life that counts, not the length.

Man is entitled to a birthright of radiant health, abundant vitality, a beautiful well-functioning body, controlled emotions, poise, serenity and self-confidence, and a free expression of the power within.

These are the rewards that come to those who practice Yoga faithfully, over a period of years. Age no longer has power over them, for Yoga is a veritable fountain of youth. It preserves and enhances the powers of man so that life can be fully lived and enjoyed as long as the body lasts.

PREPARATION FOR THE PRACTICES

The physical training of Yoga is concentrated in time, space, and equipment. No gymnasium is necessary; no tennis court nor golf course, horse, dumbbells, punching bag, nor any kind of apparatus.

All that is required is a space a little larger than the human frame, and a folded blanket or a thin pad approximately three feet by six. If a separate room is available, well ventilated and free from disturbance, it will be a great aid in practicing Yoga. Such a room is also valuable as a retreat for concentration and meditation, where the human battery can be recharged. It becomes a quiet sanctuary apart from confusion and turmoil, in which physical, mental, and spiritual strength can be found. As Whittier wrote:

> I find it well to come
> For deeper rest to this still room;
> For here the habit of the soul
> Feels less the outer world's control
> And from silence multiplied
> By these still forms on every side,
> The world that time and sense have known
> Falls off, and leaves us God alone.

HINDRANCES TO THE PRACTICE OF YOGA

Yoga should not be undertaken merely from idle curiosity, but only with a real desire to learn. Without this constructive attitude the best results cannot be obtained. In practicing Yoga, privacy and reticence are very important. The exercises are not to be exploited as parlor tricks, even for intimate friends, because personal development is often checked if the principles are indiscriminately discussed. As the *Hatha Yoga Pradipika* (one of the oldest texts on Hatha Yoga) states:

A Yogi desirous of success should keep the knowledge of Hatha Yoga secret; for it becomes potent by concealing, and impotent by expressing.

Information on the subject should be given only to those who ask for it, and who are sincerely interested. There should first be a wish to know, a certain appetite for knowledge.

It is natural to want to pass on to others what is helpful to oneself. But until through practice a true understanding of the far-reaching principles underlying Yoga has been gained, it is not possible adequately to explain or to apply the exercises to others. New ideas are convincing only as their results can be demonstrated. "One example is worth a thousand arguments."

Individual practice should not be governed by comparison with what others can do. Those who are willing to work conscientiously, step by step, toward a goal of ultimate perfection, may in the long run surpass others who apparently had better equipment to start with, but less perseverance. It is the old story of the tortoise and the hare.

On the other hand, good judgment and ordinary common sense should be used. *Each person should study and try to find out his own capacity,* for some are inclined by temperament to go beyond their strength and should guard against overdoing, while others, more phlegmatic by nature, need to urge themselves on.

The benefits of Hatha Yoga become apparent almost at once. But permanent results appear only, as in all really worth-while undertakings, after long and patient effort. Some of the traditional effects of the practice are: a strong and beautiful body, clear eyes, glowing skin, and melodious voice; a keen mind and controlled emotions; high vitality; a bright outlook on life; and a magnetic personality.

These attributes are usually thought of as belonging to the early part of life. The ancient teachings of the East demonstrate that through the practice of Yoga it is possible at any age to recapture and retain the abundant vigor and tireless health of youth.

ESSENTIAL REQUIREMENTS

To accomplish anything in life there must first be desire, then the desire must be supported by the will, and finally there must be action. It is easy to put things off, waiting for the ideal moment to begin. There is only one time—the present.

The best time for practicing Yoga is early morning when the body and nervous system are fresh and rested. If this is not possible, the exercises may be done before the noon meal or late afternoon, but never just after eating.

Yoga teaches that sloth, or laziness, is one of the greatest of all sins. Although at first it may seem difficult to find time and energy for the work, the satisfaction of accomplishment will help to overcome the inertia of the body, and the exercise period will be looked forward to as the most stimulating part of the day.

Once a beginning has been made, daily practice in itself will build moral stamina and energy with which to continue. Here habit can be an immense help, for in habit the powerful aid of the subconscious is harnessed for constructive use. To build a habit there must be frequent and regular recall. By doing the same thing at the same time every day (without fail) , a pattern is set, and reactions become automatic. Psychologists claim that it usually takes a ninety-day cycle of intensive work to establish thoroughly a new habit pattern.

> To reap a thought is to reap a deed. To reap a deed is to reap a habit. To reap a habit is to reap character. And to reap character is to reap destiny.
>
> (Source unknown)

IV

Control—the Foundation

> The person who has control over himself verily attains
> success through faith; none other can succeed. There-
> fore with faith Yoga should be practised with care and
> perseverance.
>
> —*Siva Samhita*

IN EVERY DEPARTMENT of efficient living, control is imperative. Without control man is constantly torn by his emotions, his
mind lacks organization, and he is a slave to his body's demands.

Neither the mind nor the emotions can be adequately directed
until physical control has been established. Therefore, Hatha
Yoga begins with the training of the body so that it may become
an efficient instrument for the use of the self within. This is accomplished by certain postures (*Asanas*), whose chief aim is to
bring the body under conscious control.

The postures have several very definite purposes: they are specifically designed to stimulate and strengthen the inner organs and
nerve centers; to reverse the cycle of certain life processes, thereby
arresting the tearing down or destructive forces; and finally to
quiet the body in preparation for advanced mental work.

Before the body can be intelligently directed in action, it must
first of all learn the art of nonaction, or relaxation. We live today

under such strain that it is of vital importance to be able to relax completely. Few people know how to let go throughout their entire body. Nearly always some small, often unsuspected, tension remains. No one thing, perhaps, can better help us to stand the pace of modern living than the ability to release tension.

The first posture in Yoga is called the Corpse or Death Posture (*Mritāsana* or *Savāsana*) . The body must "die" in order to be born anew. In complete relaxation it becomes as inert as a corpse.

When the body has been trained to this complete relaxation it is then ready to learn how to produce the right kind of tension. Conscious, directed tension comes through the practice of the postures, which are intended to be held for some time without moving.

HOLDING THE POSTURES

Holding a posture in complete stillness is more difficult, actually, than strenuous exercise. But there is more to be gained through this holding in stillness than from most outer forms of activity. There are several reasons for this.

First, by holding the postures the muscles are gradually stretched to their full length, from bone to bone, causing the blood to flow evenly through without strain. In this way long and graceful muscles are developed, those of all-round efficiency rather than those that furnish power in limited areas only, such as a prize-fighter's biceps. Muscular limitation can be overcome more quickly through the practice of Yoga postures than by any other form of exercise.

Second, by holding the postures pressure is developed which creates heat, stimulates the nerve centers, and increases the circulation of the blood. The entire body is evenly toned up, without sudden violent motions or jerks. There is no exhaustion following the practice, in fact quite the contrary: the body is recharged with vitality, ready and willing to carry out the orders of the mind.

Third, by holding the postures concentration is developed. Few people are intelligently aware of their physical functioning. Holding the postures gives the mind time to become centered in the body. Deliberate control is established, and there is a conscious directing of all physical functions.

It is much easier to be active than to be still. Most of us have small automatic habits, such as frowning, blinking, or scratching, and we are seldom entirely quiet. These habits always indicate a leakage of energy. When they are unconscious it is usually a sign of encroaching old age.

To really hold a posture, perfect stillness is essential. Every part of the body must be motionless, and for this, mental poise and concentration are necessary. Thus the mind is trained as well as the physical instrument. A vast reservoir of energy is unlocked, raising the level of achievement far above the ordinary standard.

THE PURPOSE OF CONTROL

The outer control of the body is only a means of regulating the inner functioning. Through muscular co-ordination the glandular and nervous systems are affected. With properly controlled breathing, when the muscles are tensed circulation is increased, stimulating the nerve centers which in turn act upon the glands. Between the nerves and the glands there is constant interplay; the whole metabolism of the body can be lowered or raised by increased pressure on, or release of pressure from, the main nerve centers.

The nervous system is to the body what the mind is to the brain: the director or controller. Mastery of the nervous system directly affects the central switchboard, or the mind.

There are three nerve centers, or plexes, in the body, that are of special importance. One is located near the throat, another in the abdomen (the solar plexus) and the third near the base of the spine (the lumbo-sacral). These centers usually function in an automatic or reflex manner as part of the sympathetic nervous system, but by practice and concentration they can be brought under voluntary control to an almost unbelievable degree. This is accomplished by certain "Locks" taken in connection with the postures.

The purpose of the Locks is to gain control through the nerve centers of the entire nervous system. In some of the more advanced breathing practices the Locks are a means of holding air within the body.

Bandha, the Sanskrit word for Lock, means literally a holding in bondage. It is an intense contraction of particular muscle groups, especially effective in stimulating nerve centers. The Lock is a governor or regulator. By reflexly activating the plexes through muscular contraction and at the same time controlling the breath, pressure is created. With the breath held in, nerve reactions are stimulated and blood pressure heightened. When held out, it is lowered. This brings elasticity to the blood vessels. The Lock acts like the squeezing of a sponge. When it is released a fresh and cleansing supply of blood flows in.

The first Lock, *Jalandhara-Bandha,* is at the throat. By dropping the chin to the hollow at the base of the neck and tensing the surrounding muscles, the thyroid and other glands are stimulated and literally pour energy into the blood stream.

The second Lock, *Uddiyana-Bandha,* is at the pit of the stomach. This most important of all the nerve centers, the solar plexus, is sometimes called the second brain, or brain of the involuntary nervous system. It is also the heat regulator. Just as the sun gives heat to the outer world, so does the solar plexus to the body, hence its name. Great heat can be induced by exercising this center, thereby increasing the digestive fires, burning up excess fat, and ridding the body of carbonaceous waste products. The practice of the Solar-Plexus Lock brings extraordinary results. By reflex action it automatically stimulates other nerve centers as well, at the throat and at the base of the spine.

The third *Bandha, Aswini-Mudra,* is known as the Rectal Lock. There are many nerve centers in the rectal region. By gaining control of the muscles at this center and through tension and release stimulating the blood supply to the nerves surrounding it, the whole system can be either tensed or relaxed. Local difficulties such as hemorrhoids, relaxed vaginal and bladder muscles following childbirth (largely caused by congestion or lack of circulation) are greatly benefited by this practice.

All of the Locks are of great importance. They are used in connection with most of the postures, and should be practiced with increasing intensity as muscular control is gained.

V

The Postures

No man wishing to develop his body, mind, and soul
. . . can afford to overlook *Yogic Asanas* (postures).
　　　　　　　　　　　　　　　　—Kuvalayananda

The *Asanas* are a means of gaining steadiness of position, and help to gain success in contemplation without any distraction of the mind.
　　　　　　　　　　　　　　　　—Pancham Sinh
　　　　　　　(Introduction to *Hatha Yoga Pradipika*)

To THE UNINITIATED the Yoga Postures may seem impossi-
bly difficult and complicated. But with patience and perseverance
any normal person can learn to do the greater part of them. Even
people advanced in years, or not strong enough for other forms of
exercise, can profit by work in Yoga. It is especially fine for men
and women beyond middle life who want to keep in good condition both mentally and physically and to retain their youthful
vitality.

The Postures may be roughly divided into three classes: those
which are performed sitting, lying down, or in inverted position.

20

SITTING POSTURES

In the Sitting Postures the spine, which carries most of the burden of everyday activity, is held erect and well elongated. The chest is opened up, abdominal muscles are relieved of downward pull, and attention is focused on that part of the body where all the vital organs lie, that is, between the neck and hips. A tendency to curvature of the spine, often due to muscular spasticity and frequently occurring in those who work long hours bending over a desk, can be largely counteracted.

The Sitting Postures are especially designed to develop flexibility in the legs. The joints of hips, knees, and ankles are exercised to the utmost capacity of their structure and function, thus keeping them flexible and limber without the violent activity of running, jumping, etc.

Very few physical-culture systems use the hip joints to their fullest capacity, opening them to the side and rotating them in their sockets. These sockets often become stiff and ingrown, even in quite young people. A flat and open groin improves the general posture and appearance, and keeps the hips in proper alignment.

Ingrown hip joints sometimes cause a slight curvature of the lumbar region (sway-back), throwing the buttocks backward and distorting the general appearance. Stiffness of the hip joints can cause complications throughout the sacral plexus, where lie so many important functions, especially in women. Where this rigidity exists, the internal organs may be thrown out of position, thus impairing the circulation and causing menstrual trouble and difficulties in childbirth. In both men and women this inflexibility may be a contributing factor to one of the commonest of all human complaints, backache. Also, intestinal elimination is usually poor where there is rigidity in the hip joints.

In addition to developing flexibility in the hips, the Sitting Postures keep the knees and ankles flexible. To be weak in the knees is often an actual physical fact. The knees support most of the weight of the body and have the greatest responsibility in maintaining it upright. Because of this special strain, even athletes often have trouble with their knees. Old age is often first evident in stiff knee joints.

In the Sitting Postures the knees, relieved from the weight of the body, are strengthened so that they can do more work with greater ease and less danger of breakdown. Of special importance is the improvement in circulation to the lower limbs and spine, preventing many ailments due to poor blood supply, such as cold feet, "housemaid's knee," varicose veins, and others. The legs and thighs are kept in beautiful contour; also a greater supply of blood is sent to the sacral plexus and reproductive organs, thus overcoming congestion and ensuring better elimination.

LYING-DOWN POSTURES

The Lying-down Postures remove the weight from the bony frame. There is not even the effort of holding the spine and head erect, as in the Sitting Postures. Since the body is on a horizontal plane, circulation is equalized. There is no downward pull of gravity; the work of the heart is immediately reduced forty per cent, and the abdominal organs and thorax are freed and relieved from weight.

The Lying-down Postures are chiefly a means of stretching the spine, thorax, and pelvis. By raising the hips while lying flat and bringing the legs over the head, the body takes its first step in altering the circulation, in preparation for the Inverted Postures.

INVERTED POSTURES

Most important of all the postures are those which are performed in the inverted position.

If nature is allowed to rule, eventually the tearing-down forces will overbalance those which build up. But if we use these latter forces intelligently, they can be turned to our advantage. By temporarily altering the body's processes the destructive, or aging elements, can be arrested. Every moment of our lives certain of the cells in our body are disintegrating while others are building up to take their place. We should try not only to keep a balance between the two, but to increase the living forces.

This is accomplished to the greatest degree in the Inverted Postures. In them all Yoga is involved, for here we have the most dramatic of all reversals. Where in standing there is a natural downward pull of gravity on the internal organs, in the Inverted Postures this pull is temporarily counteracted and the internal functions are greatly benefited. Circulatory congestion is relieved thus aiding digestion and elimination and permitting the organs to operate with less effort, and the glands are stimulated.

BENEFITS OF THE INVERTED POSTURES

The Inverted Postures are particularly beneficial to the heart, for in the upside-down position less effort is required to pump the blood through the body. The venous blood with its impurities is more easily carried off, since it now flows downward from the lower extremities instead of having to be pumped back to the heart by the veins as in standing. Elasticity of the blood vessels and smallest capillaries is thereby improved, especially in the brain. This is of great importance, since many old-age diseases such as arthritis, high blood pressure, and hardening of the arteries, are in large part the result of lack of pliability in the blood vessels.

Apoplexy or stroke, usually brought on by physical overexertion, emotional strain, or tension, causes an increase in blood pressure in the fine capillaries of the brain which have become atrophied or hardened from lack of exercise. Unable to accommodate to the extra demands, they burst and hemorrhage.

The body should first be accustomed to the inverted positions through various preliminary stages. Thus gradual pressure is added to the capillaries of the brain, creating in them the elasticity necessary to accommodate to extra demands.

Occupations requiring much sitting cause a slowing down of circulation. The blood remains in the hip region instead of flowing freely through the limbs. Cold feet result, and the restricted circulation encourages a tendency to put on fat around the waist, abdomen, and hips. The Inverted Postures relieve and offset these tendencies.

Another important result is the strengthening of the muscles that support the spine, training it to proper alignment without the need for special adjustment treatments. The Head Stand is the answer to perfect posture. In this position all the ills of wrong posture can be corrected.

MAIN INVERTED POSTURES

There are three main Inverted Postures: the Shoulder Stand, the Plough Posture, and the Head Stand. Each affects specific parts of the body. In the Shoulder Stand the glands of the throat are especially benefited. The neck is a region of vital circulation, containing the jugular vein, thyroid and parathyroid glands. Here also are located the fifth and seventh cervical vertebrae, in which great nerve strain occurs in everyday work such as bending over a desk, driving a car, and many other occupations. The Shoulder Stand stimulates these regions and causes an extra supply of blood to be sent to the glands.

With advancing years, deficiency in the secretion of the thyroid gland causes a general slowing down of the system, loss of energy, and putting on of weight. Both the Shoulder Stand and the Plough Posture help regulate the thyroid by stimulating the circulation of blood to this gland. The main function of the Plough Posture, in which the feet touch the floor over the head, is to keep the spine flexible and elongated. In later life the spine becomes stiff and has a tendency to shrink. Because of lack of exercise the cartilage between the vertebrae loses its resiliency, and the vertebrae sometimes grow together. This greatly impairs the circulation to the nerve centers in the spinal column.

THE HEAD STAND

The Head Stand, by markedly altering the circulation, is highly beneficial to all the glands in the body, sending them a fresh supply of blood and removing many fatigue products from the tissues.

The Head Stand is especially helpful in counteracting brain fag. The brain needs an extra supply of blood when it does mental work. If this is lacking, fatigue results. Fatigue is usually caused by general sluggishness of the circulation or an undue tension at some point of the body. By turning upside down, faulty circulation is relieved. Improving the circulation of the brain means that more oxygen and other nutrient substances are brought to the cells and more waste products are carried away to be eliminated by the lungs, kidneys, skin, etc. This naturally improves the various functions of cerebration such as concentration, memory, acuity of perception and reaction, integration and co-ordination of thought processes.*

The Head Stand releases pressure at the base of the spine, in the sacral and lumbar regions, thus benefiting the reproductive organs and freeing them from congestion. The eyes, ears, sense of smell and taste are also improved. Colds, sinus trouble, and headache are relieved.

It would be hard to list all the advantages of the Head Stand. The present-day fad for inverted boards as an aid to beauty recognizes its value. Most of the ills of the flesh can be alleviated by daily practice of this posture. Among other things it is an excellent face lifter, and stimulates the growth of hair. There is, in fact, no practice more effective in renewing the circulation, and this is the end purpose of all exercise.

MEDITATION POSTURES

Certain of the Yoga postures have been specifically designed to still the body in preparation for controlling the mind, particularly those in which the legs are crossed. In the Crossed or Locked-Leg Postures, the supply of blood to the vital organs and nerve centers is increased.

In order to still the mind, the nervous system must be controlled. This is the first step toward quieting mental activity, and is essential to concentration. The main purpose of the Meditation Postures is not so much physical benefit as mental power. When the postures can be held with ease, combined with the Locks and controlled breathing, the mind is released from the distractions of the body and can become centered within.

Another aid in focusing the mind is to hold the gaze fixed, without straining. The optic nerve goes directly to the brain, therefore by controlling or focusing the eyes, the mind can be affected. If the eyes are held without wavering for a period of time, the outside image gradually disappears and the attention becomes transferred from the external world to the inner working of the mind.

* Toxic substances in the circulating blood, resulting from overeating, overdrinking, insufficient water, and constipation, are powerful factors impairing normal cerebration.

This can be accomplished by holding the gaze fixed to one point, not by straining the eyes (this is most important) but by gradually building up capacity through increasing the practice period. As the optic nerves and muscles are strengthened, the eyes too are benefited. Clear and sparkling eyes are an indication of health, and they also reveal character. A shifty gaze, or eyes that are never still, show mental instability and wandering wits, while a direct and steadfast gaze at once proclaims a strong character.

VI

Cleansing Practices

Cleanliness of body is ever esteemed to proceed from
a due reverence to God.

—Ruskin

THE OLD SAYING "cleanliness is next to godliness" is in Yoga
a literal and scientific truth. But here *internal* cleanliness is meant
rather than that of the surface alone. To gain lasting benefit from
Yoga practices it is necessary to maintain a standard far above the
generally accepted idea of a clean body.

At the beginning of the work the body is not always capable of
adequately carrying off waste products, such as lactic acid and
carbon dioxide, residue of muscular activity which accumulates in
the tissues and causes fatigue. Without a high degree of cleanliness
these wastes may create muscular soreness and general acidity of
the digestive tract. Hence the importance of first cleaning out the
system before undertaking the practices.

There are three products of the body that are highly detrimental
if they accumulate in excessive quantities: bile, toxic gas, and
phlegm. A sluggish liver impairs the normal flow of bile, causing
it to back up into the system and giving rise to biliousness. Toxic
gases absorb the oxygen in the system and cause a feeling of torpor,

27

while phlegm and mucus are the carrying medium of germs. Before starting the Yoga practices it is important to get rid of these, and to clean out all the avenues of elimination.

Internal cleansing does not mean going against natural functions. It means increasing the power of elimination, thereby assisting nature. Since extra demands are placed on the body in the Yoga exercises, all its functions should be correspondingly heightened.

ELIMINATION

Man's natural power of elimination has been largely lost through artificial living. A considerable part of his work is sedentary, with lack of sufficient exercise and overindulgence in food and stimulants. The abdomen is usually the least exercised part of the body. Yet it is here, in most people, that the first signs of slowing down appear. With advancing years, elimination becomes sluggish and poisons gather, fat accumulates, and there is a gradual deterioration of the organs.

The alimentary tract, from mouth to excretory organs, is called in Sanskrit *Shakta-Nadi* the power tube, because all of life is sustained within it. During its course from mouth to exit lie all the main functions of digestion, assimilation and elimination. Even the lowest forms of life have an alimentary tract. Some organisms have little else. Vitality depends on the healthful condition of this power tube, especially of the abdominal region. If no other part of the body could be exercised but the abdomen, it would still be possible to maintain health.

Perhaps the greatest single handicap of modern man is inadequate elimination, and its attendant autointoxication. The same blood circulates through the brain that flows through the intestines. If the bowels are lazy, the entire system becomes sluggish, the brain is dull, and the spirits depressed. A good cure for the blues is to clean out the intestinal tract.

Greater attention, actually, should be given to elimination than to what is put into the system. But the reverse is usually true. We are more concerned with stoking the furnace than in cleaning out the clinkers. Yet the fires of energy can never burn with a bright flame if they are smothered with ashes or waste products.

If the simple elements of nature, such as water, fresh air, and sunshine are utilized, together with the Yoga work, it will soon become unnecessary to resort to drugs and medicine. Colds, congestion, catarrh, fever, infectious diseases, skin eruptions, and many other ailments could be largely prevented by the simple expedient of keeping the colon free of unnecessary waste matter.

INTESTINAL CLEANSING

One of the best ways to maintain health and prevent disease is to flush out the intestines regularly, not by the use of purgatives, but with water.

In the original Yoga practices centuries ago, cleansing the colon was accomplished by squatting waist deep in water while alternately contracting and releasing the abdominal muscles and by this means creating suction and drawing water into the bowels. Before expelling the water certain abdominal exercises were performed, in order to churn the intestines and thoroughly clean them out while still squatting in the water.

This type of colon cleansing (*Basti*) requires a high degree of muscular control. Equally beneficial results can be obtained today with an ordinary enema when taken in connection with abdominal exercises.

The enema has been criticized as unnatural and habit-forming. If used alone, without the special exercises, the colon might in time become weakened and grow flabby and lazy. But if the enema is performed with a proper understanding of the structure and function of the intestinal tract, and always in connection with certain of the Postures and abdominal exercises, then instead of being weakened the muscles are strengthened and built up, and a normal habit of elimination can be established even though it may never have existed before.

The Yoga abdominal exercises provide an internal massage of the most efficient sort; they tone up both the exterior and interior muscles, and prevent conditions, such as prolapse of the stomach, uterus, and other vital organs, and general lack of tone of the intestinal muscles (with flaccidity and spasticity) which causes constipation.

These exercises also have an important effect on the solar plexus, that great nerve center which regulates the involuntary automatic functions of the body. They increase the peristaltic functions of the bowel and stimulate the digestive juices and secretions of the liver, pancreas, and gall bladder.

As a result, digestion and general assimilation are improved, excess abdominal fat is eliminated, the circulation throughout the body is increased, the blood stream purified, and the skin becomes fresh and clear. In short, abdominal exercises assist and stimulate all of nature's functions.

OTHER AVENUES OF ELIMINATION

The kidneys, skin, and lungs are all organs of elimination, and should be kept scrupulously clean. So should the openings of the body: the nostrils, ears, eyes, mouth, rectum, and vagina.

The kidneys can be cleansed by drinking plenty of water, preferably between meals and several glasses at a time. This extra intake of water helps to dissolve the waste products so they can be carried off by the kidneys.

Another means of elimination is through the skin, by perspiration. Copious perspiration, which can be induced by exercise, clears out clogged pores and helps the skin to breathe and regenerate itself. It also takes some of the burden from overworked kidneys. The lungs likewise help to rid the system of impurities, notably of carbon dioxide.

Air and heat are used as well as water in purifying the body through Yoga methods. A number of the exercises generate heat at the solar plexus, the fire center of the body. Deep breathing creates internal heat and aids digestion. Externally, sunshine is of great value as an asepticizer and purifier. Certain beneficial properties inherent in the rays of the sun can be absorbed through the skin. Regular sun baths, if not carried to excess, are helpful to the system as a whole.

AIR AS A CLEANSER

Air is especially important as an aid in cleansing the system. Deep breathing aerates the body and carries oxygen directly to the blood stream. By deliberately swallowing air with water, in connection with some of the abdominal exercises, peristaltic action is increased, helping to push food along its way and preventing constipation.

The early Yogis observed that certain animals are great air swallowers. Birds, for instance, make themselves light by swallowing quantities of air. Those that eat carrion flesh are especially given to air swallowing, a practice which helps to purify their systems and keep them from getting poisoned. Bears also, before hibernating, fill themselves up with air. Snakes take in quantities of air to aid them in digesting the animals which they swallow whole.

Purification should be the first step in the physical practice of Yoga. When the body is clean and free of impurities, and under control, then it is ready to start work on the postures.

VII

Prana, the Breath of Life

> When Prana moves, the mind also moves. When
> Prana ceases to move, the mind becomes motionless.
> . . . Therefore one should control Prana.
>
> Mind is the Master of the senses, and the breath is
> Master of the Mind.
>
> —*Hatha Yoga Pradipika*

P*RANA* IS A Sanskrit term that has no real equivalent in other
languages. It has been translated as vital energy or life force.
Prana, like electricity, exists in essence all around us; it is in the
air we breathe, the food we eat, in water, and also in sleep. Whatever inspires us is likewise a source of this subtle, life-giving element. Our words inspiration and spirit both come from the Latin
spiro, which means breath.

An old Chinese proverb says: "Consciousness is like a kite;
breath the string that guides it." The ancient Yogis discovered
that by control of the breath, heightened states of awareness could
be attained.

Breath is our most important link with *Prana,* and is the chief
means by which this vital force may be taken into the body. The
new-born infant comes to life with its first gasp of air, and life

departs with the last breath drawn, leaving the body heavy and inert.

Since breath is the medium of consciousness, in order to be more alive and in every way more alert, we should use more breath. It has been said: "He who only half breathes only half lives."

In ordinary breathing one fifth or less of the lung capacity is used. The average person takes in just enough air to keep life functioning. When special demands are made, as in running or any unaccustomed exercise or emotion, the body has great difficulty in meeting the emergency. The heart beats like a trip hammer, trying to pump more oxygen into the blood, the pulse runs wild, and sometimes the fine capillaries of the brain burst, as in apoplexy.

Rhythmic, directed breathing offsets the wear and tear of life. Through regulated breathing exercises the entire circulatory system is stimulated and toned up, keeping it flexible and as a result able to accommodate to strain and emergency. Like a tree in the wind, it bends but does not break.

Air is not only indispensable to life but more essential than either food or water. We can live for days without nourishment, but only a few minutes without oxygen. This vital element is the greatest purifier that exists; it stimulates, cleanses, repairs, detoxifies, and asepticizes the impurities of the body. Breath is the principal means by which oxygen is brought into the blood stream and carried to the nerves and brain.

In everyday activity we use up all the oxygen that we take in. Deep breathing increases this intake, and likewise quickens the elimination of carbon dioxide gas. When the breathing is shallow, residual air with its load of carbon dioxide remains in the lungs like water in a stagnant lake. Daily exercises in aerating the nasal and lung passages help to prevent coughs, colds, and sinus trouble.

AIR CONDITIONING

In the pioneer days of flying, aviators discovered that breathing exercises were of great importance in training them to adapt to high altitudes and to the strain that flying brought to ears, lungs, and other parts of the body. Pearl divers, who remain under water for several minutes at a time, have learned the value of controlled breathing. They "air-condition" themselves through special exercises, going through a definite routine before diving, emptying the lungs and then filling them to full capacity. On coming out of the water they let the breath out very slowly before resuming normal breathing.

We have become very air conscious in modern times. But although we recognize that air is more important to us than any other element, we have concerned ourselves more with air-conditioning our houses than in air-conditioning our bodies.

THE MAGIC SHORT CUT

Breath is the magic short cut to all exercise. If a person has physical limitations that make ordinary exercise impossible, certain of the less strenuous Yoga breathing practices can still be done with benefit.

Breathing can also be the most vigorous form of exercise. In order to gain the advantages of its power, however, it is imperative to have a well-functioning, thoroughly clean body, for otherwise the stimulation of deep breathing may stir up existing impurities in the blood stream.

On first taking a really deep breath there is sometimes a sensation of dizziness, but this is only because the system is unaccustomed to so much oxygen. The temporary giddiness passes as the body develops greater capacity for accommodating larger quantities of air. There is nothing physically dangerous about such symptoms, nor should they be confused with psychic manifestations. Effects produced by *physical* causes have too often been mistaken for *psychic* phenomena.

At first *lung capacity* is the principal aim of the breathing exercises. The beginner should be mainly concerned with getting as much air as possible in and out of the lungs, in order thoroughly to aerate and open them up, increasing the expansion of the rib cage and at the same time strengthening the thoracic muscles.

Only when this has been accomplished can *control* of the breath be attempted. Through this control of the breath eventually comes control of the mind and the senses.

CONTROL OF THE MIND THROUGH BREATH

Mental states are closely reflected by the breath. In excitement breathing is fast and erratic, uneven and disturbed. In depressed moods there is a limited intake of air and much outgo, as in sighing and shallow breathing, while in moments of calm the rhythm of the breath is so silent as to be almost imperceptible. When the mind is in a state of acute attention or intense concentration, the breath is actually momentarily suspended. Concentration in its purest form can only be maintained as long as the breath is held.

In the same way that breath is affected by the mind, so the mind can be influenced by the breath. Everyone goes through periods of emotional crises that seem almost unendurable, such as acute pain, anger, or grief. If in these moments of distress quiet, rhythmical breathing is practiced, it will greatly assist in maintaining, or even in restoring, equanimity. When accidents occur, one can often retain consciousness and prevent fainting by becoming aware of the breath through watching its ingoing and outgoing.

In any emergency or strain there is no greater support than deep, sustained breathing. Control of the mind through the breath can even render the body insensitive to pain.

Pranayama, or training in breathing, focuses the mind, helps to control the emotions, and calms the nervous system. It is the first step in meditation: the key that unlocks the gates to wider consciousness.

THE SCIENCE OF SOUND

Closely related to the science of breath is *Mantra Yoga,* or the science of sound as it affects man's inner forces. A *Mantra* is, literally, a phrase or formula used to influence the subconscious with the significance of its truth. Such a formula possesses great creative power. The first manifestation of creation was through the spoken word. The opening phrase of the Gospel according to St. John states "In the beginning was the Word."

The basic *Mantra* of the East is a rhythmic repetition of the word OM (or AUM) which, it is believed, liberates consciousness.

If one wishes to impress any fact or truth on the mind, there is no more effective means than by repeating, over and over again, a phrase that suggests the idea. In recent years great emphasis has been laid on the value of autosuggestion: impressing the subconscious through spoken or mentally repeated formulas. This is an everyday use of the power of *Mantra*.

Sound influences the emotions as well as the mind. Strident, martial tunes arouse combative instincts, while soft, harmonious melodies have a soothing effect even on the mentally disturbed. Noble music lifts men's souls and fills them with inspiration. All religions make use of this principle, recognizing the power that lies in chanting, singing, and prayer.

Prayer, a form of *Mantra,* can be either spoken or silent. Silence, the great primeval void, is latent sound—the womb from which sound springs.

SOUND AS SPEECH

Speech is our chief means of communication with others. The voice, which is the physical medium of speech, is a sure indication of the personality within. People are often more affected by this attribute of character than by any other outward expression.

The quality of the voice also reveals the emotional state. A harsh voice is not only unpleasant to hear, but it actually brings about unhealthy reactions within the body of the speaker. If we become aware of a jarring quality in our own voices, we should recognize it as an indication that something is wrong. It usually means that we need to train our bodies to more harmonious functioning. A low voice, sweet and clear, should be consciously cultivated; for in the same way that a harsh voice brings destructive reactions, so a pleasing voice is health giving.

The Yoga practices give depth and a vibrant quality to the speaking voice, notably the Humming Breath, which utilizes the constructive power of sound, causing vibration through the entire mechanism of the body and mind.

The breath should always be kept under control; in this way energy is conserved. A silent man is usually master of his emotions. Conversely, the garrulous person not only exhausts the breath of life but is emotionally uncontrolled. Since speech (that is, sound) is power, it should be used intelligently and not needlessly dissipated for trivial purposes. We of the West are not sufficiently aware of the great power of properly directed sound.

> Four things are necessary in practicing *Pranayama*. First, a good place; second, a suitable time; third, moderate food, and lastly, purification of the *Nadis*.
> —*Yoga Tantra Samhita*

VIII

Diet, Relaxation, and Sleep

> From the time he begins till the time he gains perfect
> mastery, let the Yogi eat moderately and abstemiously;
> otherwise, however clever, he cannot gain success.
> —*Siva Samhita*

To OBTAIN the best results in Yoga, it is important to guard
against overindulgence of any appetite, whether it be eating, sleeping, smoking, or any form of intemperance.

Eating should be primarily a means of replenishing the body.
Elaborate meals of rich and highly seasoned foods load down the
system and place great strain on its working mechanism, causing
general sluggishness and often resulting in functional disorders.
To digest unnecessary food, large amounts of energy are required.
Energy can be put to better purposes.

After the body is cleaned out and in perfect working order, unnatural cravings and wrong habits will no longer appeal. When
assimilation is improved, less food is needed. It is an excellent plan
to give the digestive system an occasional rest, and to skip a meal
if tired or run-down or emotionally disturbed. Eating when fa-
tigued or without appetite not only burdens the body with more
work but poisons the system as well. An occasional twenty-four

hour fast can be helpful.* During such a fast plenty of water should be taken, at least two glasses every other hour, and there should be extra rest and a cleansing of the bowels.

Raw foods, fruits, vegetables, milk, and whole-grain cereals should be an important part of the regular diet. The general inclination is to eat too much fat and oil, sugar and starch. These foods have a tendency to produce acid and mucous conditions. The natural sugar in fruits and the starch in whole grains and certain vegetables are preferable for the body's needs to any processed foods.

In a healthy state the body's tissues, blood, etc., are slightly on the alkaline side. Much disease could be avoided by the simple expedient of maintaining this alkaline balance. If there is sluggishness from poor elimination, the body cannot throw off excess acids. Mucus and overacidity accumulate in the stomach and intestines and frequent colds result, together with an increased susceptibility to current epidemic diseases, due to the lowering of the body's natural resistance or immunity factor.

Alcohol, like sugar, is acid forming and has a tendency to burn up the oxygen in the system. It acts like a whip, momentarily stimulating the body's functions. But as with all stimulants, the temporary lift is usually followed by a corresponding letdown. While the body can tolerate small amounts of alcohol it must not be forgotten that alcohol is classified as an intoxicant, and this means that excessive amounts are toxic, or poisonous.

PROTEIN AS ENERGY BUILDER

The most important of the three energy-producing elements is protein. Protein, among other vital compounds, supplies a necessary organic form of iron for the blood which has the capacity of combining with the oxygen in the lungs. A certain amount of this organic iron is required to keep us from becoming anemic. When we are anemic we have no stamina, tire easily, get out of breath, have muscular cramps, and become nervous and irritable.

* After the system has been thoroughly conditioned by the Yoga practices, it is possible to obtain added benefit from a three- to five-day, or even longer fast. A singular state of lightness, mental clarity, and general well-being will result.

THE VITAL IMPORTANCE OF WATER

It is most important that there should be sufficient intake of water. But it is best not to drink it with meals, since this dilutes the digestive fluids. Too much salt in the diet causes excessive retention of fluids in the tissues of the body. The average adult should excrete about a quart and a half of moisture in twenty-four hours, and to do this there should be a fluid intake of at least two quarts, since about a pint is lost in evaporation from the breath and in perspiration. Various conditions, such as climate or kind of work being performed, may modify this ratio a little, but this is the average norm.

Why is it necessary to drink so much water? Chiefly because various end products of food digestion, particularly those from protein, must be eliminated or they become toxic to the system through reabsorption. With too little water these end products are not sufficiently diluted to go into solution so that the kidneys can excrete them. In high-protein reducing diets it is particularly important to drink plenty of fluids.

Water taken in adequate quantities also acts as a laxative. No other fluid takes its place. The best time to drink is between meals, when there is no food in the stomach. By drinking several glasses at one time the whole system is cleaned out and impurities are carried off by the kidneys. At least two glasses should be taken every morning before breakfast. Before retiring, however, it is better not to drink, since the water tends to place an extra burden on the kidneys and the heart. This is especially important for anyone who is trying to reduce, as water taken just before retiring is absorbed during the night and adds weight. The liquid content of the body is over eighty per cent of the total weight.

VITAMINS

Vitamins play an important role in the proper assimilation of food, the maintenance of correct muscular tone, balance of the glands, metabolism, and so forth.

Unfortunately, much of our food today is deficient in vitamins. Farmlands have been depleted by overproduction and failure to replace minerals taken from the soil, while the food grown on them often lacks the normal supply of vitamins. Cattle and poultry fed with synthetic foods are apt to produce milk and eggs low in vitamin-giving elements. The refining of grains and sugar and the processing of fruits in canning and freezing, destroy some of these elements so imperative for healthful living.

Vitamins alone, however, cannot correct dissipation of the body's forces by wrong habits of living, eating, lack of proper exercise, and insufficient rest and relaxation. On the other hand, scientific exercise can so raise the metabolism that wholesome food will of itself alone furnish all the necessary elements.

THE RELATION OF MIND AND EMOTIONS TO DIET

A tense, high-strung temperament prevents the proper assimilation of food. Nervous indigestion caused by worry, hurry, or general tension is a common symptom of modern life. The mental and emotional attitude of the individual has too often been overlooked in the matter of diet. The condition of the mind at the time of eating has great influence on the body's power of digestion and assimilation.

Disappointment, frustration, or overexcitement often create reactions that unconsciously seek satisfaction in overeating or in loss of appetite. The excessive craving that is sometimes felt for food or drink is often no more than a hangover from an emotional jag. Most cases of obesity have only one real cause: overeating. Self-control should regulate our eating habits.

There are no hard and fast rules for diet. The rate of metabolism and chemical balance varies in different people. The main thing is to know one's personal idiosyncrasies and then to use common sense. Eat simple, wholesome food, in small quantities at regular, well-spaced intervals. If this regime is carried out and the general principles herein described are followed, together with the Yoga practices, a high standard of health and well-being can be established and maintained.

SLEEP

Efficient living demands a balance between the active and the passive. Nature demonstrates this principle: action is always followed by its reaction—rest. Night succeeds day; winter follows summer; after the drawing in of breath comes the outgoing exhalation. Even the heart itself has its fractional moment of complete rest between the systole and diastole.

In order to gain the utmost from any form of activity, we must balance it with its opposite, rest. The greater the pressure, the more necessary it is to learn how to let go. Tension long continued defeats its own purpose, efficiency becomes impaired and relaxation impossible. Overfatigue and nerve exhaustion will prevent sleep, with its natural recuperative powers. It is impossible to sleep well if there is tension, either mental or physical.

When the body is trained through Yoga to function properly and control is gained both of the outward vehicle and the inward direction, then tension can be released normally by conscious relaxation and restful sleep comes naturally.

The Relaxation Posture is of special help in counteracting tension just before going to sleep. When in bed, an invariable habit of quiet and calm should be cultivated. If sleep will not come, instead of tossing restlessly about it is better to get up, stretch, and do rhythmic breathing and relaxation exercises. A few minutes lying flat on the hard floor will make the bed seem soft and comfortable by contrast, and sleep usually follows.

Tension is one of the greatest obstacles to restful sleep and, in fact, to general well-being. Today people are resorting more and more to "peace-of-mind pills." Through drugs, tranquilizers, or stimulants, the nervous system is either whipped up or let down. We are coming to rely more on pills than on our own will power and strength of character.

Unfortunately, the more we resort to artificial aids, the weaker we become and less capable of meeting the adverse elements in our environment. It requires effort and courage to live. Life is a constant challenge; if we fail to grow and unfold we die—slowly or quickly, partially or completely, in one or all three planes of existence, physical, mental, or spiritual.

TOO MUCH SLEEP

While a sufficient amount of rest is very important, there is such a thing as too much sleep. A sluggish system resulting from overindulgence in food, lack of exercise, and general wrong habits of living, induces drowsiness. Sleep can be a drug or opiate which the subconscious suggests as an escape from the problems or boredom of life. This usually comes from a failure of the conscious self to face difficult situations. Complete understanding of a problem, facing it realistically in all its various aspects and then acting decisively, dissolves that problem once and for all, making it unnecessary to waste energy by continuously battling the same difficulty.

Sleep has an overpowering influence on the mind. With the approach of night the body undergoes certain changes and an entirely different rhythm is established. However, the nervous system should be so trained that if necessary one can go without sleep or food, for there are times of emergency when it is of vital importance to stay awake and be in possession of all one's faculties.

OTHER MEANS OF REPAIR

Sleep is not the only means of repairing the body. When it is essential to remain awake and mentally alert, breathing exercises and additional food are helpful. Deep breathing is an immediate recharger. The Head Stand also helps to restore energy, and so does meditation. Meditation is akin to deep, dreamless sleep; it has even greater recuperative powers.

When one is very tired, a few moments of conscious relaxation will often be found more restful than sleep. Relaxation brings many benefits. It gives one a sense of perspective, and in times of emergency it is invaluable. The relaxed person puts others at their ease, and in every situation will get better results than one who is tense or in any way disturbed.

Directed relaxation, or intensity without effort, brings one to the central point of perfect balance where achievement far beyond the average becomes possible. The ideal state is one of effortless skill, such as is found in the highest expression of creative artists.

Life, with its sunshine and shadows, should be the conscious experiencing of a wonderful adventure.

IX

Sex

We are apart, that we may learn the Way together
That way to blessedness in each other's hearts
That symbolizes that blessedness at Home with Thee.
May we aspire apart to form together one great cup
In the fullness of days upheld for Thy fulfillment.
                                                    —W. Comfort

THE PRACTICE of Yoga develops and increases every faculty of a human being, and it lays special emphasis on the right use of the sex force. This most vital medium of creative energy is recognized as an evolutionary power, to be treated with profound respect as a means toward man's greatest potentialities.

A well-integrated human being usually has a strongly sexed nature. High spirits, good appetite, a keen enjoyment of life, all indicate that this force is present. So-called "goodness" is sometimes lack of sex power rather than a virtue. On the other hand, a real saint may be as highly sexed as a libertine; the difference between the two is a matter of control and direction of the underlying force. Nothing influences character more than one's attitude toward sex.

Today we are surrounded on all sides, through advertisements, literature, and so forth, by stimulants with so-called sex appeal, which overemphasize the physical aspect of this basic force. Having put aside our natural instincts, we are less controlled than animals, and because we do not know the right use of sex we unknowingly and needlessly dissipate our vital energy.

Of all man's attributes, sex is the one that has been least understood. Its physical expression is but the outward form of an inner power that is literally the mainspring of all creative activity. Passion is the "wind in our sails." Before we can direct our ship we must have this force to impel it; as with all energy, there must first be capacity, then control, and finally right direction.

The only way that sex can be controlled and intelligently directed is through an understanding of its true nature.

THREE WRONG USES OF SEX

There are three wrong uses of sex: abuse, nonuse, and overuse. Under the first heading come all the perversions which violate the laws of nature and have a destructive effect on the personality. These perversions are merely sex substitutions; the natural relationship cannot be transcended. The second way, nonuse, if wrongly understood can be almost as harmful to the individual as overuse, though the latter is perhaps most injurious of all, since it dissipates so much creative force. Overindulgence in the physical expression of sex depletes the entire nervous system and undermines the character as well as the physical stamina, so that in time even the power of indulgence is lost. Don Juan is the classic example.

All religions have recognized the value of control and discipline in sex. This has been one of the most important means of training for spiritual consciousness. Overindulgence has always been preached against, although it is actually less of an offense against morality than a violation of one of nature's fundamental laws.

Complete asceticism, on the other hand, can also be destructive. Where it becomes fanatical, or restriction is imposed arbitrarily from without, energies are merely dammed up and more harm is done than good. But when restraint is practiced wisely, great power can be gained. This restraint, however, must be *voluntary*, a matter of personal choice rather than an outwardly imposed restriction. The practice of asceticism is really a misunderstanding of continence. Continence means a willing foregoing of momentary gratification for the sake of greater eventual gain. Intelligent, that is, purposeful continence hoards sex power instead of expending it all on the physical plane. In this way tremendous energy can be accumulated, ready for use on other creative levels.

DIFFERENT ASPECTS OF SEX

In a well-balanced, normal man or woman, sex is expressed not through one channel alone, but in every aspect of life. If physical expression is denied to people of this temperament, they will find other ways of using their sex force instead of losing themselves in the conflict and frustration that so often comes to those who understand sex only from the physical side.

Too much emphasis has been laid on the necessity for a physical experience of sex. Even where complete abstinence is practiced, it is possible to live without detriment to health. Man functions as much on the mental plane as on the physical. If his general outlook is sound, and if he realizes that the great force of sex may be used in other ways than the physical, he can become master rather than slave of this compelling impulse.

Sex includes many factors. Love, loyalty, devotion, self-sacrifice, all play a large part in its full expression, and have tremendous power in developing creative force. We cannot adequately function on the physical side alone, for if we deny our emotions and seek only a casual physical release, we do violence to our noblest capacities.

Love possesses the magic power of heightening all of our faculties and lifting us to new regions of understanding and achievement. Even when unrequited, it exalts and quickens the consciousness. Witness some of the famous loves of history—among them Dante and Beatrice, Héloïse and Abélard, Tristan and Isolde.

For most people, however, the greatest fulfillment is reached through a happy, harmonious relationship between man and woman, where both know the right use and expression of sex and have a common basis of understanding and cooperation. When there is a mutual aim toward higher realization, both gain immeasurably from such a partnership, and each develops a capacity for advancement beyond what is possible through separate effort.

The *Kama Sutra,* an ancient Indian scripture, lists the following stages of Love:

1. Receiving
2. Exchange
3. Love unrequited
4. Love as fulfillment of the Law
5. Temporary loss of self
6. Recognition of oneness of love expressed by two: "Where each is both."

Yoga teaches a way to use sex force intelligently, whether on the physical plane or in other creative ways. As man raises his spiritual powers to a higher level he will find less need for, yet more to be gained from, the physical experience of sex. Eventually, when there is a well-integrated relationship and both partners in the sex act have equal understanding and high purpose, the outward expression becomes a communion engendering spiritual power, a sacrament consciously directed toward higher realization.

X

Mind Power and Meditation

To that man of high aim, whose body, mind, and soul
act in correspondence, the higher, nay even all the
secrets of nature become revealed. He feels within
himself, as everywhere, that universal life wherein
there is no distinction, no sense of separation: yet all
bliss, unity, and peace.

Yoga Sutra of Patanjali

ALTHOUGH Hatha Yoga is primarily concerned with the
physical side, its main objective is to control the mind, which in
turn opens the way to higher consciousness.

We of the West have been inclined to use mind power chiefly
for material benefits. Because we are a practical race, we have concentrated on worldly matters and have paid little attention to
spiritual development. On the other hand, without sound physical
equipment, spiritual research can bring disturbance to both mind
and body. The imagination may take control and pose as reality,
creating illusory phenomena that, while often pleasant and exciting, have no real value. True spirituality is far removed from
physical and psychical manifestations.

Since we in the West are by nature an active race, achievement
for us must come mainly through action. According to Yoga phi-

losophy our present era is called the *Kali-Yuga* age, and has as its keynote "realization through action." Therefore Hatha Yoga, with its emphasis on action, is not only the way best suited to Western temperament, but actually the one most fitted at this time to lead man to ultimate self-realization, a state as far beyond our present limited understanding as the human world is from that of the animal.

All of life is but a preparation for this realization; in fact the Eastern sages, who believe that man must continue to pursue life experience until he is awakened to an understanding of his real purpose, claim that it takes at least three lifetimes of constant, sustained endeavor to make a Yogi.

THE VALUE OF PERSISTENCE

No effort is ever wasted, but we will naturally reach the goal faster if our work is sustained. Progress does not move forward in a continuous line. It proceeds in a series of irregular steps, with long intervening plateaus between. At times we may feel that we are moving forward with swift, well-directed purpose, then a longer period follows when no progress seems to be apparent and we doubt if we shall ever reach the goal. Discouragement, however, if rightly understood should act as a spur to greater effort, and if we persist we will soon take another step forward.

The long, level plateaus of apparent nonachievement might be likened to a period of gestation, necessary before further advance can take place. Understanding this law helps to make the seemingly sterile periods less depressing.

MIND CONTROL

Everyone realizes the importance of a well-trained mind. All of life should be used for this training. By giving our entire attention to whatever we do, no matter how trivial, and becoming completely absorbed in it, we help to develop mind control. A mind trained to concentrate is like a burning glass, kindling to fire whatever it may direct the sun's rays upon.

There are definite exercises in controlling the mind, just as in controlling the body. By practicing these exercises, "mental muscles" can be built up which will be found useful in all thinking.

As preparation for this work the physical functions should first be quieted; then directed, rhythmic breathing should take place and finally a conscious focusing of the mind. Eventually it will no longer be necessary to go through each of these steps. As concentration grows into a habit, the powers of the mind will become so strengthened that every thought or problem serves as material, and mental force can be turned on without effort.

The exercises in mind training should, whenever possible, be performed in one of the Postures especially designed for this purpose. The Meditation Postures hold the body in complete stillness, so that its demands are reduced to a minimum and the mind is free to concentrate.

Control of the mind brings an inner tranquility that has far-reaching effects on every part of human existence. Poise, discrimination, harmonious adjustment, equanimity in every experience —these are some of the results of this way of life.

EXERCISES IN MIND CONTROL

The initial exercise in mind control is mainly to relax the mind from all tension. The first part, watching the breath, can be practiced at any time with benefit.

I. Reflection—*Pratyhara*

Sit in one of the Meditation Postures. If this is not yet possible, then take any sitting position in which the body is held erect with the spine in perfect alignment.

First spend some time in rhythmic breathing. Try to make the breath progressively calmer and more even until, as the old precept says, "A feather held under the nose will not be stirred." When a feeling of deep tranquility has been reached, then turn the attention within and watch the thoughts go by as in a passing show. Do not try to focus the mind on any particular idea or problem, but simply see yourself as a spectator.

This detached observation, watching the body, emotions, and thoughts, is the first step toward a release from their demands. One of the most important by-products of the practice of Yoga is an impersonal attitude in considering the different aspects of the self, and particularly of the body. Eventually this impersonal viewpoint becomes second nature and one begins to realize that the physical vehicle is only the instrument of the self within.

By quietly examining the thoughts that come, you will recognize, and eventually discard, a great deal of useless mental activity, such as day dreaming and superficial speculations. Unless these idle thoughts or waste products of the mind are eliminated, they will continue to disturb and distract. Watchfulness acts as a mental purge and is an important preliminary to meditation.

II. Concentration—*Dhāranā*

When the above holding of the mind has become possible, select some object and consider it closely, in every detail. Anything will serve, such as a flower, photograph, or person. Then close your eyes and reproduce the image mentally, keeping the mind firmly fixed upon it. If the mind wanders, as it is sure to do, direct it again to the object under consideration. A means of keeping the mind focused is to fix the gaze on one point and hold it there steadily. This practice is known as *Trātaka*.

The next step is to replace the object by some ideal or abstract virtue. This has value from a character standpoint, for "we are shaped and fashioned by what we love."

When concentration is complete, the whole being will be focused not on, but *in* the object or ideal. All thought of self or separation will be lost. One becomes a part of the essence of what is contemplated. This is called Absorption.

III. Contemplation—*Dhyana*

After the mind has learned obedience in holding to the one in the many, then the third step can be taken. In this stage all the forces of the mind are directed to an imaginary center.

The breath, as in all of the meditation practices, should remain calm, even, and unhurried, until with complete concentration it becomes temporarily suspended.

When *Dhyana* has been perfected, the self is liberated from its limitations and merges with the Absolute Reality, or pure consciousness, the source of all existence. This state is known as *Samadhi*.

THE SEVEN CENTERS

According to Yoga there are seven centers of psychic energy, called *Chakras* or wheels, that have relative counterparts in the human body. These are located at the base of the spine, at the sacral center, the solar plexus, heart, throat, between the eyes, and at the top of the head. By awakening these centers, man's evolution can be hastened.

When both the physical and the mental practices have been brought to a high degree of perfection, the student may be qualified to begin the advanced training of the seven centers.

At the lowest of the *Chakras* lies a latent power called *Kundalini*. This creative force can be aroused and directed upward through the various centers, awakening each in turn and eventually reaching the highest, where it becomes united with spiritual power. The training to animate this force, however, is only for the serious and advanced student who, after years of patient and persevering practice, has reached a high state of proficiency and is privileged to study under the direction of a competent teacher.

The Meditation Postures, together with mind and breath control and the exercises in concentration, are a necessary preparation for this advanced work.

There is no end to Yoga. In this book only a beginning has been indicated. But it is a beginning of great importance, for physical control is a means to mental and spiritual achievement.

Part II—*The Technique*

The Technique

THE FOLLOWING INSTRUCTIONS for the various Yoga practices have been prepared with great care. They are explicit in every detail, and if the directions are carefully followed, step by step, it should be possible even without the help of a teacher and with no previous training or special aptitude, to obtain remarkable results.

Before beginning any of the work in Yoga it is important to spend a few moments in relaxing the entire body.

Relaxation Posture—*Savāsana,* or *Mrilāsana*—known as the Corpse Posture

1. Lie flat on the floor.

2. Draw several long, deep breaths, and *let go in every part of the body.*

To relax completely it is helpful first to gradually tense the entire body, hold this tension for a moment, and then let go—completely. Think successively of the different parts of the body: the hands, feet, legs, trunk, head, neck, and throat, and particularly the mouth and eyes, making each part progressively heavier than the last. Then let the body slowly melt away, until it feels light as air.

55

Complete relaxation is reached when the body has apparently ceased to exist.

Note. It is helpful to take this Relaxation Posture not only at the beginning, but at intervals during the other exercises, or at any time in the day when one is tired or conscious of tension. At such times it is not necessary to lie down. Perfect relaxation can be achieved in any position, at any time, when once the technique has been learned.

PREPARATORY EXERCISES

Since the physical practice of Yoga requires a suppleness far beyond the average, it is wise to prepare the body—through a few preliminary exercises—in order to start the circulation and to overcome stiffness in the muscles and joints. Few people in the West are equipped at the outset to do the Postures in their original forms. But with certain modifications and an initial limbering up through the following preparatory exercises, it is possible eventually to become proficient.

THE STRETCHES

Stretching is nature's way of rousing sleeping cells. It starts the blood flowing more rapidly in preparation for action. Animals use this principle. They never dash into activity; when they first wake from sleep they shake and stretch themselves, and become fully conscious in every part of their bodies before attempting any activity.

Stretching is one of the best and simplest of exercises for gently stimulating sluggish circulation. This helps to carry off toxic accumulations and gives the body fresh energy.

Whenever you are tired, stretch!

1. Lie flat on the back. Relax, with arms over the head, and stretch all over.

2. Stretch up with the right arm, fingertips reaching for the opposite wall. At the same time stretch down with the right heel (*not* the toes) until the back tendons of the leg feel a strong pull. Bring right arm back to the side, then relax and stretch up with

the *left* arm, down with the left heel. Repeat both sides, always relaxing completely between stretches.

3. Now stretch up with the *right* arm and down with the *left* heel. This creates a cross or diagonal pull that should be strongly felt in the abdomen and the lumbar region of the spine. Relax and repeat with the *left* arm and *right* heel.

4. Draw up the knees and bring the hands, with fists clenched, to the shoulders. Then push up against strong resistance with both fists, gradually opening the hands and finally extending the fingers. At the same time slide the heels down, also against resistance. A strong pull should be felt throughout the body at the end of this exercise. Relax and repeat.

Suggestions for Practice

In practicing the stretches try always for a greater pull, and for more complete relaxation between the various stages. When stretching both arms and both legs simultaneously, try at the same time to press the small of the back down, and the shoulders as well. The back of the neck should also be pressed to the floor.

In this position, one is assuming—while lying down—what should be the perfect posture when standing: the head, neck, shoulders, spine, hips, and knees being in proper alignment.

When doing the stretches and, in fact, all of the exercises, the breath should be watched with great care. It should never be hurried or strained, but always smooth and under control. Do not pant or breathe through the mouth. In fact one should never be out of breath. This is very important.

CORRECT POSTURE

Correct posture is of the utmost importance. When the body is improperly held there is considerable strain on the vital organs, and this offsets much of the benefit of any exercise. To check up on posture, stand sideways in front of a mirror and draw an imaginary line through the ear, center of neck, shoulder, hipbone, knees, and ankles. The head should be pressed back against the spine so that the ears are in line with the shoulders—neither in front nor in back of them.

The abdominal muscles must not be allowed to sag. Stretch up and out of the hips and lift the rib cage to make room for the internal organs. *Never slump!* Aside from appearance, slumping is very bad for all of the organs, preventing their proper functioning and interfering with their blood supply.

THE SPINE ROCK

This exercise is especially good as a warmer-upper, accustoming the body and circulation to variations in position and movement. By rocking back and forth on the spine, the vertebrae and nerves along the spine are massaged and stretched. This increases the circulation throughout the body, and irons out the kinks in the spine.

1. Sit cross-legged, grasping the toes palms down, the right foot with the left hand, the left foot with the right hand. Bend the trunk forward as far as possible without lifting the buttocks from the floor.

2. Rock back on the spine and over onto the shoulders, bringing the feet to the floor over the head, while still keeping the hold on the feet.

3. Rock forward again to the original position, maintaining the grasp of the feet and using them as a lever in pushing forward and down. Repeat this rocking backward and forward several times.

When it is possible to do this exercise with ease, then the following, progressively more difficult stages, may be undertaken.

Variations of the Spine Rock

A. Spine-Rock without grasping the feet

Instead of holding the feet, clasp the hands together and swing them forward to the floor as you go down, then back over the head as you rock onto the shoulders.

B. Spine-Rock keeping the legs straight

Touch the hands to the toes when coming forward, and again when the feet are over the head.

C. Same as A, but after rocking back to the shoulders, rock forward and rise to a standing position, the feet still crossed at the ankles. Then return to the cross-legged sitting position and rock back again to the shoulders.

Be sure to lean the trunk well forward in rising and in returning to the sitting position. This is especially good practice for balance, and for strengthening the knees and reducing the hips.

Suggestions for Practice

All through the Spine-Rock exercises, the back should be kept well-rounded and the knees close to the chest. The closer the legs are folded against the body, the easier it is to make the rock smooth and even. It is important to feel each vertebra as it touches the floor. The body should be thought of as round, like a ball.

LEG FOLDING

Following are a number of special exercises for limbering up the legs as a preparation for the Sitting Postures. Most people have stiff knee, hip, and ankle joints. We of the West are not accustomed, as the Orientals are, to sitting in the cross-legged position. Therefore, it is especially important at the beginning of the practice to work with these joints and train them to pliability. The following preliminary leg-folding exercises are done chiefly in lying-down position, with the upper body relaxed and the spine straight and flat, so that full concentration can be focused on the stretching and bending of the joints.

1. Lie flat on the floor. Bend the left knee with foot turned outward. Then grasp the left instep with the left hand and fold the leg backward to a position beside the left hip. Press the knee and leg down to the floor until a strong pull is felt in the muscles on top of the thigh (the so-called Charley-horse muscles).

2. Straighten the left leg, then bend it in the opposite direction, outward and open. Now grasp the left foot with the *right* hand and place it on top of the right thigh, as high up in the groin as possible. With the other hand press the left knee to the floor until a strong pull is felt.

3. Straighten the left leg, then bend it back toward the chest, knee bent. Clasp the hands just below the knee and press the knee close to the chest.

4. Lift the leg straight into the air, at right angles to the body. Clasp the hands under the thigh and pull the leg toward the chest,

keeping the knee straight. Return the extended leg slowly to the floor.

These four steps should then be repeated with the *right* leg.

Variations of Leg Folding

A. Leg-folding in sitting position

1. Sit erect with both legs extended in front. Continue as in No. 1 of last exercise.

2. Same as No. 2 of last exercise.

3. Grasp the inside of the right heel with the right hand, palm downward, and extend the leg forward and up until both knee and arm are straight. Repeat this extension several times, each time returning the foot to the groin. Then lower the leg to the floor in slow extension, maintaining the grasp on the heel and keeping the body erect. Repeat with the other leg.

B. Knee limbering

1. Kneel and sit firmly on both heels, knees close together and feet under the buttocks, spine erect.

2. Slightly lift the hips and sit to the *right* of the heels, close to the feet.

3. Again lift the hips (as little as possible) and return to the first position.

4. In the same way sit to the *left* of the heels. Complete the exercise by returning to the first position.

C. "Making the Square"

1. Sit as in last exercise, arms crossed over the chest or folded above the head. Lift the hips slightly and this time push the *feet* from under the hips to the right side.

2. Extend the legs directly in front on the floor, knees straight.

3. Bend the knees sharply back and bring the feet close to the *left* side of the hips.

4. Lift the hips slightly, push both feet under them and sit on the heels as in the first position.

Note. Throughout this exercise be careful not to move the hips from side to side, as in B. Change the position of the *legs* only, keeping the hips as a center.

Suggestions for Practice

In the last two exercises be careful not to lean forward from the hips, but feel the pull at the sides, from the waistline.

Do not lift the hips *high;* only enough to tuck the feet under them.

Do not collapse as you sit, but move always in an even, smooth manner, thus maintaining control of the weight at the hips. It may be necessary in the beginning to use the hands as a help to press the hips up from the floor.

For an additional stretch from the waist, the arms may be crossed above the head, hands locked over the elbows throughout the exercises.

THE LOCKS

(Bandha or *Mudra)*

The Locks are especially designed to augment the benefits of the postures and breathing practices. By contracting the muscles of the three important plexes, at throat, solar plexus, and rectum, and at the same time holding the breath either in or out as indicated, an internal pressure is created that produces a highly stimulating effect on the nerve centers located in these regions, and vitalizes the entire nervous system.

The Solar-Plexus Lock is the most important of the three. When this lock has been perfected, the other two—at throat and rectum—automatically follow, although each may be practiced separately to acquire proficiency, and for specific results.

Wherever the Locks can be used in connection with the postures, it is mentioned in the detailed descriptions of the exercises.

A. The Solar-Plexus Lock—*Uddhiyana-Bandha*

1. Forcibly contract the abdominal muscles, drawing them up under the diaphragm and back toward the spine.

2. Relax and repeat. (See Plates 46 and 49)

The most vital and essential benefits of the physical Yoga work are obtained through the practice of the Solar-Plexus Lock. It must be developed to a high degree of proficiency before the more advanced practices can be achieved.

The Solar-Plexus Lock may be taken with the lungs empty (breath out, as in certain Postures) or with the lungs filled (breath in, as in the breathing practices). This Lock affects both the other Locks, and should be practiced whenever possible in connection with the various postures.

B. The Chin or Throat Lock—*Jalandhara-Bandha*

1. After forcibly swallowing several times in succession, contract the muscles of the throat and press the chin firmly into the jugular notch. Hold during the suspension of the breath.

2. Relax and take several normal breaths.

The purpose of this Lock is to prevent the air from rising upward, causing undue pressure on the small capillaries of the brain and sometimes bringing sensations of dizziness, ringing in the ears, etc. It should be practiced whenever the breath is suspended.

In connection with the Chin Lock it is an additional advantage to take the Tongue Lock *(Khecari-Mudra),* which is done by turning the tongue upward, toward the soft palate, and pressing it firmly against the roof of the mouth.

C. The Rectal Lock—*Mula-Bandha*

1. Forcibly contract the anal sphincters while simultaneously contracting the abdominal muscles.

2. Hold, then relax.

The Rectal Lock can also be done in the following manner:

D.

1. Take knee-chest position (on the elbows and knees). Exhale vigorously and take the Rectal and Solar-Plexus Locks with vigor.

2. Hold until a suction is felt in the rectum and abdomen.

3. Release both Locks and inhale. Repeat the contractions and relaxations several times.

This practice is known as *Aswini-Mudra.* It can be done in almost any position. When practiced in the Head Stand it is most effective in ridding the intestinal tract of toxic gases, and gives immediate relief to the uncomfortable pressure and pain caused by these gases.

The purpose of the Rectal Lock is to strengthen the muscles surrounding the anal sphincters so that they may be controlled at will. In the advanced practices the Rectal Lock is used to draw air and water into the intestines for cleansing purposes.

This Lock may be practiced to advantage in most of the Sitting Postures, including the Back-Stretching (Plate 8) and Meditation Postures (Plates 32–35). In the breathing practices it should always be combined with the Solar-Plexus and Chin Locks.

THE SITTING POSTURES

Exercise *within* the trunk of the body, where all the vital organs lie, is the chief objective of the Yoga Postures. These are performed chiefly in seated, lying-down, and inverted positions.

There are several reasons for this. One is economy of force. By taking the weight off the feet, the maximum results are obtained with a minimum of energy. Few people stand correctly at best, and exercise done with wrong posture cancels out most of the benefits otherwise to be obtained. (See directions for Correct Posture, pages 57–58.)

Daily activities and most physical-culture exercises are done chiefly in a standing position, which involves a certain amount of effort in maintaining the body erect. The muscles holding the organs in place, particularly those of the abdomen, have to work against the pull of gravity.

In the Sitting Postures great attention must be given to maintaining the upper body in perfect alignment. The spine should be held erect and elongated upward, the head high, the ribs lifted and opened. The shoulder blades should be flat, pressed down and backward, the chin and abdomen held in.

I. Half Posture—*Virāsana*   Plate 1

1. Sit erect, folding the left leg backward beside the left hip.
2. Place the right foot in the left groin, as high up as possible. (See Plate 1)
3. Hold and take the three Locks (Chin, Solar-Plexus, and Rectal).
4. Relax and repeat, reversing the position of the legs.

Suggestions for Practice

It is most important to keep the trunk erect and both knees on the floor. Also the buttocks should remain on the floor.

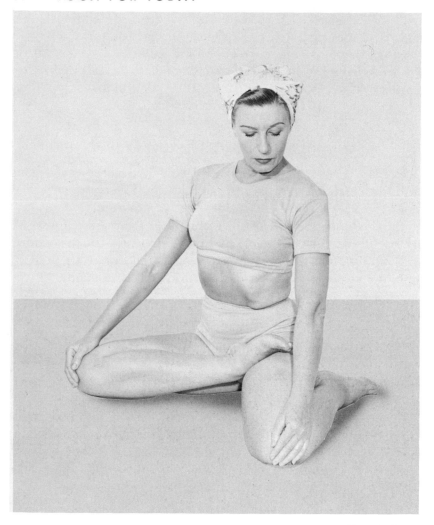

PLATE 1

This posture combines two ways of folding the legs. One side of the pelvis is opened, the other closed. The practice of the Half-Posture is a splendid preparation for the more difficult Pelvic and Lotus Postures. It has special value as an exercise for flexibility in the hips.

II. "V" Posture—*Samkatāsana*   Plates 2 & 3
    1. Sit with the legs extended in front.

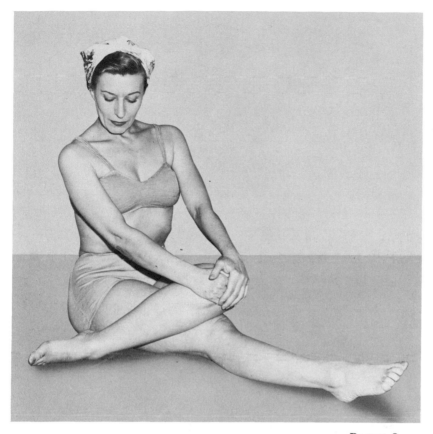

PLATE 2

2. Bend the left knee and place it on top of the right thigh, bringing the leg close beside the right hip. (See Plate 2)

3. Bend the right leg under the left thigh and bring it close to the left hip. Place the hands palms down on top of the knees and press them to the floor. (See Plate 3)

4. Hold and take the three Locks. Then relax and repeat, reversing the position with the right knee on top of the left.

(See Variations, pages 132–133)

Suggestions for Practice

The hips should be firmly touching the floor, the spine held completely erect, and a strong tension maintained throughout. Do

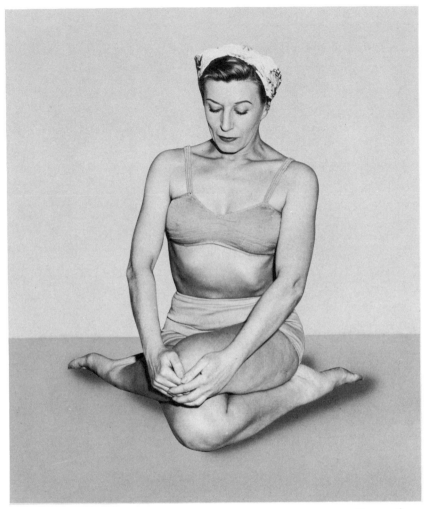

PLATE 3

not relax at any point. Try to bring the legs as close to the thighs as possible.

The purpose of the "V" Posture is to create heat through tension. This is effected by bringing the knees close together and pressing them to the floor with the arms extended. By maintaining the posture with strong tension, a trembling of the entire body will be felt. This stimulates the nervous system. Special flexibility of the knees is required in this posture.

III. Frog Posture—*Mandukāsana*   Plate 4

1. Sit on the heels in a squatting position, keeping the knees, heels, and toes together.

2. Fold the arms at the chest, or over the head, clasping the elbows. (See Plate 4)

3. Hold the posture and take the three Locks.

(See Variations, pages 133–134)

Suggestions for Practice

Keep the spine straight, and do not lean either forward or backward from the waist. The weight should be kept well back over the heels, in line with the spine, the hips touching the heels.

PLATE 4

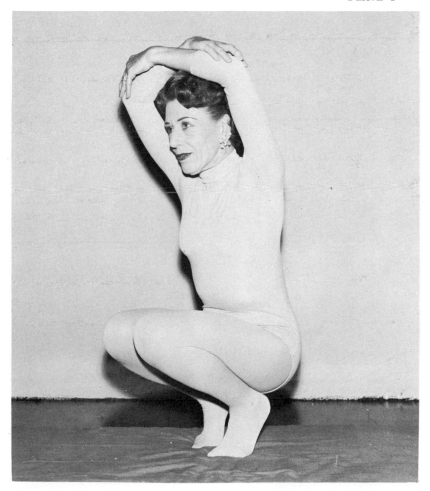

This posture is especially good for strengthening the muscles that support the arches of the feet. It helps fallen arches and so-called flat feet. It is particularly effective in developing balance.

IV. Crossed Posture—*Bhadrāsana*   Plate 5

1. Kneel and sit on the crossed feet, right ankle over left, right heel pressing up into the perineum.

2. Fold the arms across the back at the wrists, right arm under left, and grasp the toes of the left foot with the right hand, the right toes with the left hand. (See Plate 5)

3. Hold the posture and take the Chin Lock.

4. Relax and repeat, reversing the position (left ankle over right, and left arm under right).

PLATE 5

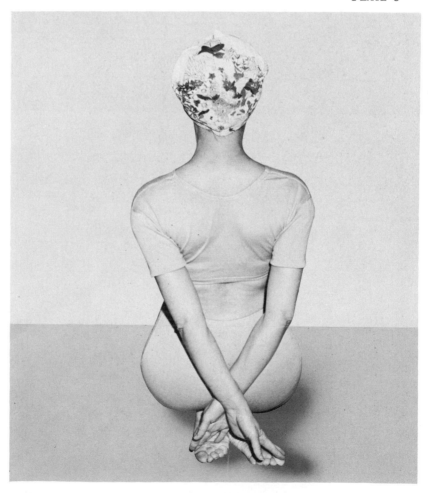

Suggestions for Practice

Do not lean back, as this will make the spine arch and the stomach protrude.

Keep the knees together and the thighs touching the floor.

If at first you find it difficult to grasp the toes, practice clasping the hands behind the back and pulling the shoulders open and down, gradually stretching until the feet can be reached.

This posture opens the chest, lifts the ribs, stretches the diaphragm, and forces the shoulders back and down. The upward pressure of the heels on the perineum is beneficial in stimulating elimination of the bowel, by offsetting the downward and outward pressure. It also brings about better circulation to the perineum.

The pressure and weight placed on the ankles reduces excess fat and helps to keep the ankles trim.

V. Spine Twist—*Ardha Matsyendrāsana*   Plates 6, 7

1. Sit with the legs extended in front. Place the left foot flat on the floor to the right side of the right thigh. Bring the left knee to the chest.

PLATE 6

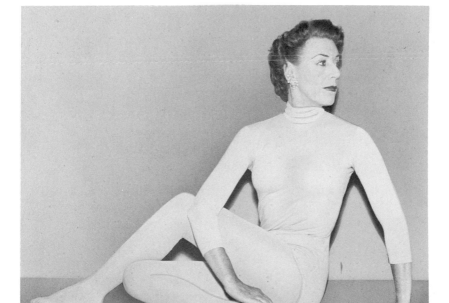

2. Bend the right leg at the knee and bring it back, close beside the left thigh.

3. Twist the waist to the left until the back of the right elbow can be hooked over the left knee. (See Plates 6 and 7)

4. Grasp the left heel with the right hand, placing the left hand on the floor at the back, in line with the shoulders. Turn the head far to the left.

5. Repeat on the opposite side.

(See Variations, page 134)

Suggestions for Practice

Keep both hips firmly on the floor, and the trunk erect.

Do not bend forward. Tension should be felt from one end of the spine to the other and throughout the body in order to create

PLATE 7

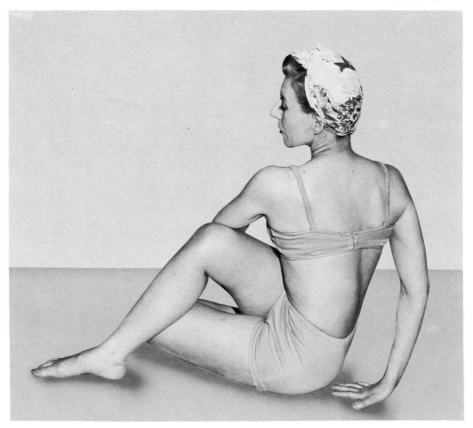

the necessary pull. If the head or chin come forward the pull is broken.

A strong cross-pull of the spinal column is brought about in this posture. The sacral and lumbar regions are pulled in opposite directions, as well as the cervical and dorsal. This creates great flexibility in the spine; and releases impingements or tensions of the nervous system. It is also beneficial in slimming the waistline.

VI. Back-Stretching Posture—*Paschimottanāsana* or *Padhahasthāsana*   Plates 8, 9, 10

1. Sit with legs extended in front, knees straight.
2. Bend forward from the waist and grasp the toes without bending the knees or lifting legs from the floor. (See Plate 8)
3. Still keeping the legs straight, bring elbows to the floor and the head to the knees. (See Plate 9)

PLATE 8

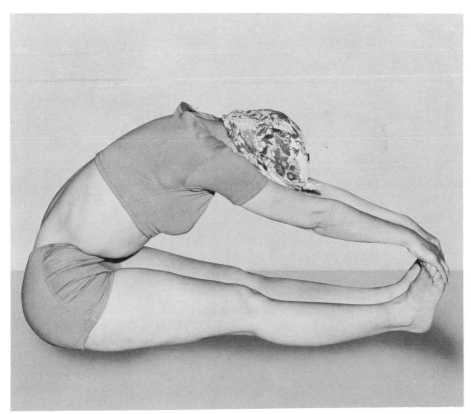

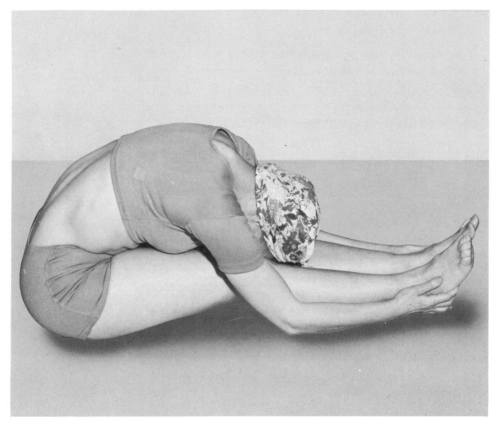

PLATE 9

4. Hold the posture and take the three Locks.
(See Variations, pages 134–135.   Plate 10)

Suggestions for Practice

It is most important to keep the knees straight and as flat on the floor as possible.

The second step, bending forward and grasping the toes, must be practiced until it becomes easy before continuing with the third step (bringing the elbows to the floor and the head to the knees). At the beginning if it is too difficult to reach the toes, the ankles may be grasped instead.

In this Posture the three Locks can be held to particular advantage.

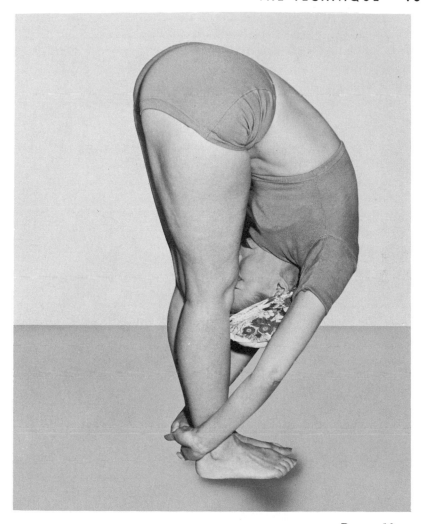

PLATE 10

The main purpose of the Back-Stretching Posture is to stretch the spine and to open up and separate the vertebrae. It elongates the muscles on both sides of the spine and helps to prevent the compression or shortening of the spinal column, which usually occurs with advancing age.

Although this posture is especially intended for the spine, it is also very good for the back muscles of the legs (known as hamstrings) and helps to relieve cramping and knotting of the muscles in the calves and thighs, and maintains them in symmetrical contour. In addition, the Back-Stretching Posture is excellent for lifting the abdominal muscles into proper position, particularly when used in combination with the Solar-Plexus Lock. It flattens and reduces the abdomen.

Paschimottanāsana means literally: making the body like "a stick bent in two."

VII. Locked Posture—*Maha-Mudra*   Plate 11

1. Sit on the floor with both feet extended.
2. Place the heel of the left foot against the perineum.
3. Bend forward and grasp the heel of the right foot with both hands, head touching the right knee. (See Plate 11)
4. Take the three Locks with the breath held *out*.

Repeat with the opposite leg extended.

Suggestions for Practice

If at first it is difficult to grasp the foot, hold the ankle instead.

Both legs should be flat on the floor, the chest touching the thigh.

PLATE 11

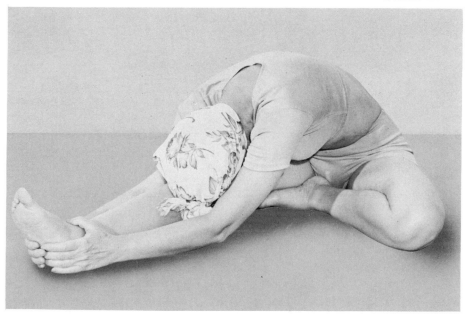

In this position the benefits of the Back-Stretching Posture are combined with pressure on the abdomen, by placing the heel against the perineum. This posture is always combined with the three Locks. Its purpose is to bring air high into the lungs, thus opening those parts of the chest seldom reached by ordinary exercise. The pressure also creates internal heat.

VIII. Pelvic Posture—*Vajrāsana*   Plate 12
  1. Kneel and sit between the legs.

PLATE 12

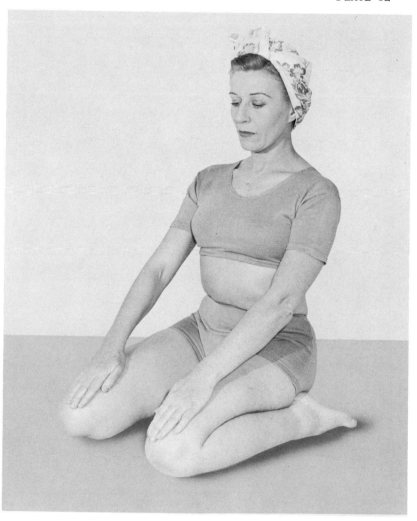

2. Fold the lower legs back against the hips, knees either together or partly open. The insteps may be flat on the floor, or slightly turned out. The arms may be extended forward with the hands grasping the knees, or crossed over the head. (See Plate 12)

3. Hold the posture and take the three Locks.

(See Variations, pages 135–137.   Plates 13, 14)

PLATE 13

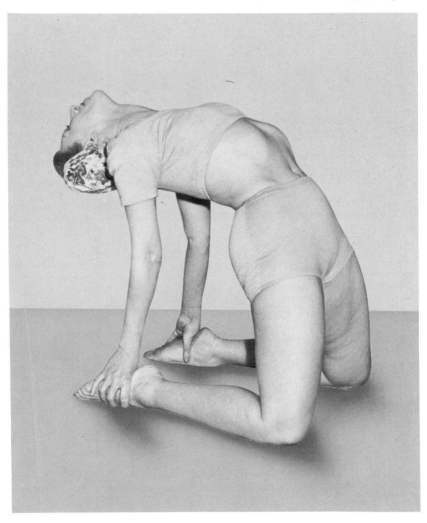

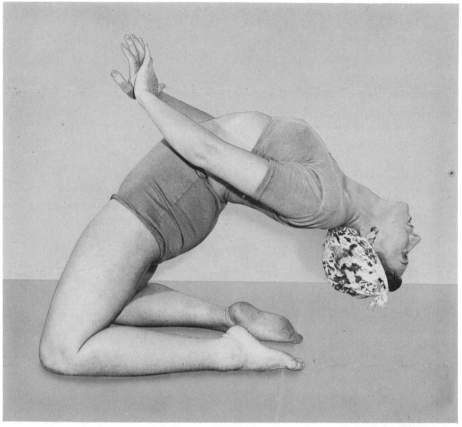

PLATE 14

Suggestions for Practice

The posture should be kept as compact as possible. Do not spread the legs out, but keep the feet close to the thighs. The knees may be either closed or open, and the buttocks should touch the floor. This exercise is also called "sitting between the hips."

In the Pelvic Posture the thigh muscles in the front of the legs (sometimes called Charley-horse muscles) are lengthened and strengthened, reducing fat in the hips and thighs. It is one of the most important exercises for developing flexibility in hips and knees.

IX. Supine-Pelvic Posture—*Supta Vajrāsana*   Plate 15
 1. Take the Pelvic Posture. (Plate 12)
 2. Lean back from the waist, gradually lowering the spine until you lie flat on the floor between the legs. The arms may be placed on top of the thighs palms down, crossed over the head, or extended upward. (See Plate 15)
 3. Hold the posture and take the three Locks.
(See Variations, pages 137–139.   Plates 16, 17, 18)

Suggestions for Practice

In the beginning this posture may be done by placing the hands palms down on the floor beside the feet and then dropping the weight on the elbows and lowering the back until it touches the floor.

PLATE 15

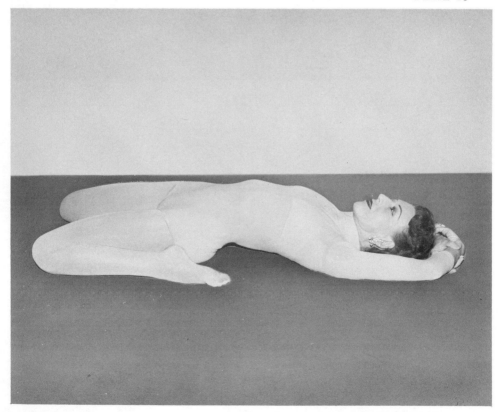

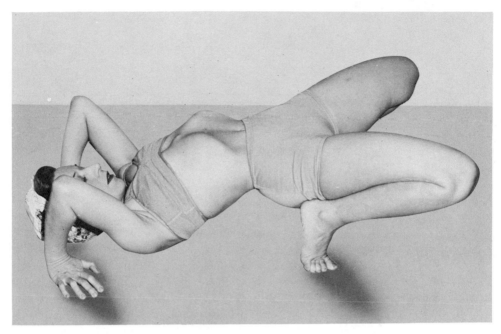

PLATE 16

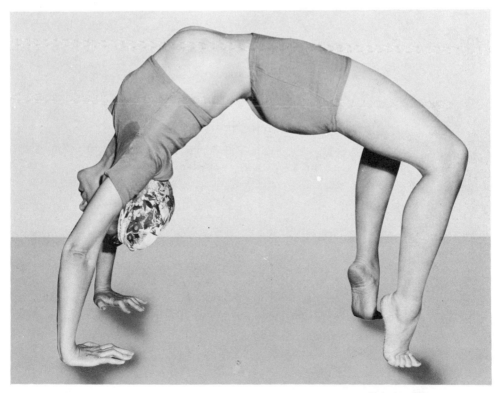

PLATE 17

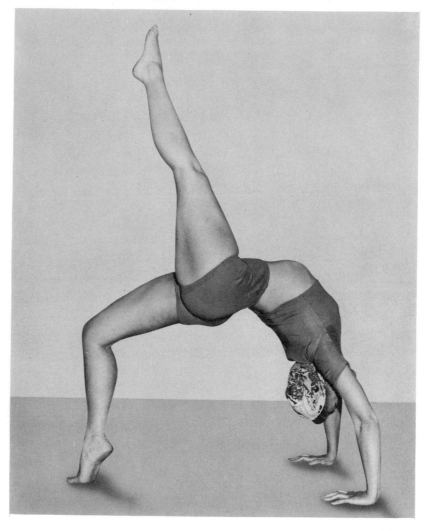

PLATE 18

A strong pull in the muscles of the thighs and abdomen is felt in this posture. It opens the pelvis and groins and frees the organs in the abdominal cavity.

LYING-DOWN POSTURES

X. Cobra Posture—*Bhujangāsana*   Plate 19

1. Lie flat on the abdomen, forehead touching the floor.

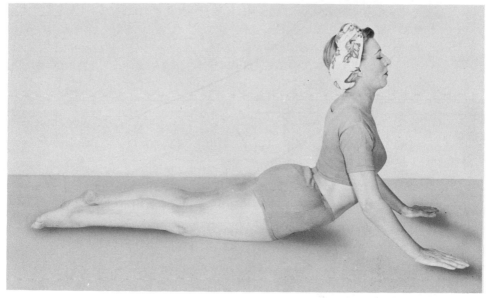

PLATE 19

2. Place the hands at the shoulders about three feet apart, elbows straight, shoulders back and down.

3. Press the body up from the hips, arching backward without lifting the hips from the floor, the legs remaining straight and together. (See Plate 19)

4. Hold and take Chin-Lock.

(See Variations, page 139)

Suggestions for Practice

Arch back from the waist only, keeping the abdomen flat on the floor.

For the beginner it is permissible to have the legs slightly apart, making it easier.

The Cobra Posture (so-called because of its resemblance to a cobra with head raised, ready to strike) is especially good in correcting maladjustment of the spine. It develops the deep muscles of the back, so seldom used in ordinary activity, stretches the spine and makes it flexible, and opens the shoulders and chest.

The sympathetic and autonomous nervous systems, and indirectly the brain, are stimulated by this exercise.

XI. Locust Posture—*Salabhāsana*   Plate 20

1. Lie on the abdomen, arms placed closely at the sides, the chin and chest touching the floor.

2. Press the palms of the hands down, arch the back, lifting the legs up from the hips.

3. Hold

(See Variations, pages 139–140)

Suggestions for Practice

Raise the legs from the hips as far as possible by pressing down with the hands.

Keep the legs extended and the chin touching the floor.

The Locust Posture gives the appearance of a locust, or grasshopper, with legs folded at the side and tail raised at an angle to the ground. While the Cobra Posture strengthens the upper or dorsal region of the spine, this uses the muscles of the lower or lumbo-sacral region, and the back of the legs from knee to buttocks. It is also strengthening to the pelvis and the abdominal organs.

PLATE 20

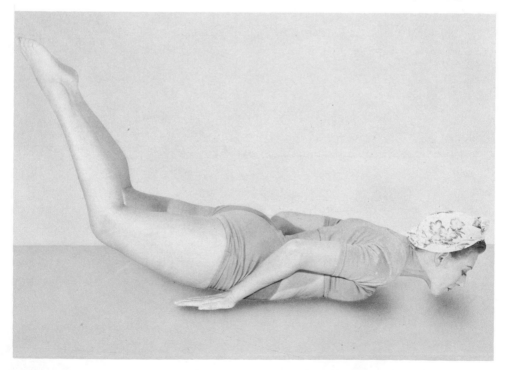

XII. Bow Posture—*Dhanurāsana*   Plate 21

1. Lie on the abdomen.

2. Bend the knees and extend the arms backward, grasping the toes or ankles and arching the back. (See Plate 21)

3. Hold.

(See Variations, page 140)

Suggestions for Practice

The thighs should be lifted as far from the floor as possible. Rocking back and forth in this posture is a good abdominal reducer. It also stretches the muscles at the front of the thighs.

The Bow Posture, in which the body resembles a strung bow, combines the effects of both the Cobra and the Locust Postures, producing a complete arch of the spine.

PLATE 21

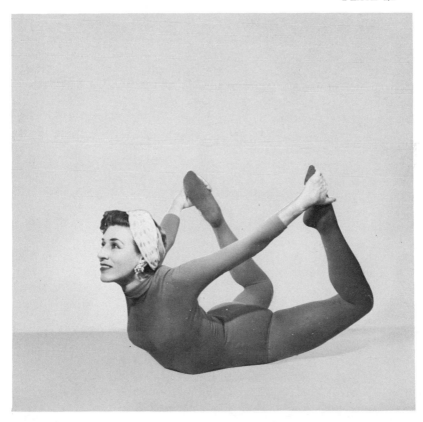

XIII. Spine-Balance Posture—*Vajroli Mudra*   Plate 22

1. Sit with the legs extended, hands on the floor beside the hips, palms down.

2. Lift the legs up as high as possible, balancing on the end of the spine. The hands should slide forward, pressing against the floor, arms straight. (See Plate 22)

3. Take the three Locks and hold.

(See Variations, pages 140–141.   Plate 23)

Suggestions for Practice

The head should be held straight on the spine, chin in.

Hold the legs as straight as possible, not bending the knees.

PLATE 22

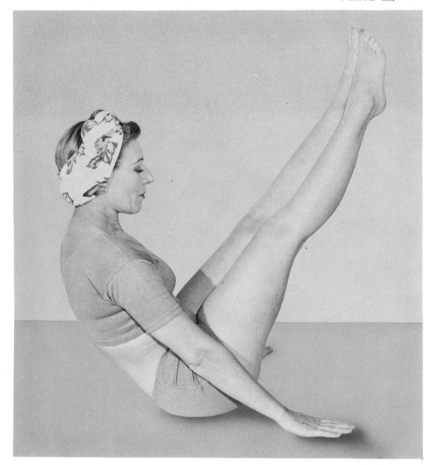

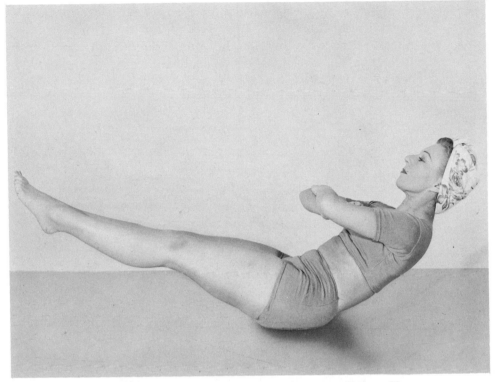

PLATE 23

The main purpose of this posture is to develop tension, which in turn creates heat, especially in the abdominal and sacro-spinal regions.

INVERTED POSTURES

The benefits of the Inverted Postures can hardly be overestimated. For the many advantages to be gained, see Chapter V.

Any new skill is difficult to master, and this is especially true where a new kind of balance is involved. The body should be *gradually* accustomed to an upside-down position.

XIV. Shoulder Stand—*Sarvangāsana*   Plate 24

1. Lie flat on the back, arms at the side, palms down.
2. Raise the legs, then the hips, and finally the shoulders, until the body is at right angles to the floor.

3. Place the hands at the small of the back, keeping the elbows close to the sides and pushing the hips forward.

4. Stretch up with the legs, the hips, shoulders, and spine in a straight line, and the chin pressed against the chest in the jugular notch. (See Plate 24)

(See Variations, pages 141–142)

Suggestions for Practice

The legs should be kept straight, the buttocks tucked in and

PLATE 24

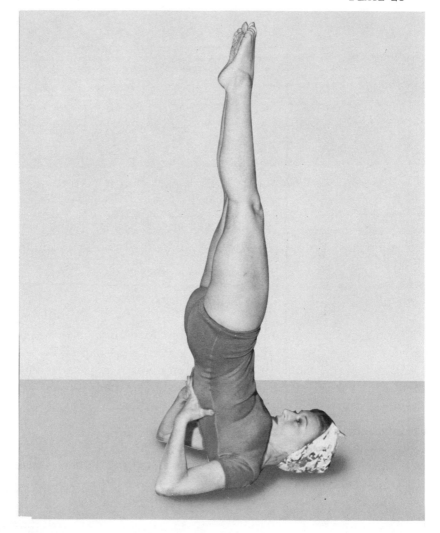

forward, so that the body is completely straight with no angle at the hipline.

Balance on the shoulders only, keeping the back completely off the floor.

Do not use the hands any more than necessary to raise the weight of the hips and to maintain balance.

The Shoulder Stand has the special advantage of pressing against the thyroid, a gland in the throat which is important to all of the endocrine system, and especially helpful in governing metabolism. The thyroid is a vital factor in health. When properly functioning it controls weight, furnishes energy, wards off old age, and affects the sex glands.

Another benefit of the Shoulder Stand lies in inducing deeper breathing. By forcing air out of the upper-lung cavity, the breathing switches from the chest to the abdomen.

The Sanskrit name of this posture: *Sarva,* meaning the whole, and *Anga,* the body, indicates its importance to the entire system.

The Shoulder Stand is sometimes called the Pan-Physical Posture.

XV. Plough Posture—*Halāsana*   Plate 25

1. Lie flat on the floor, arms at the side, palms down.

2. Raise the legs to a right angle position, keeping the arms down.

PLATE 25

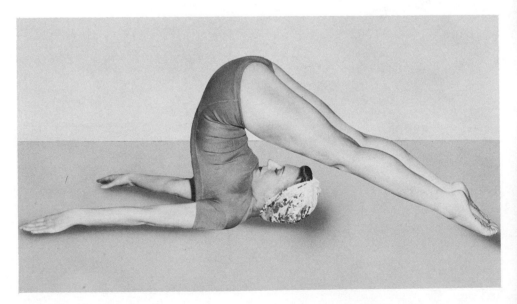

3. Lift the hips and bring the legs over the head until the toes touch the floor, the arms remaining flat with the palms down. (See Plate 25)

4. Hold.

(See Variations, pages 142–143.   Plate 26)

Suggestions for Practice

After touching the toes to the floor, continue to push them further, as a plough making furrows. The arms, flat on the floor, form the handles of the plough.

The entire exercise should be done smoothly, without jerks.

In old age, the spine tends to become rigid. The Plough Posture helps to keep it flexible. The Plough Posture also affects the thyroid gland, as in the Shoulder Stand.

PLATE 26

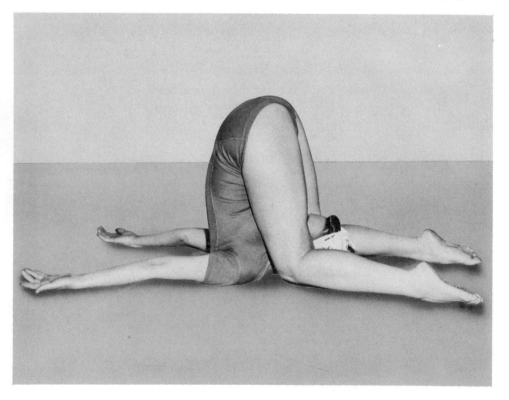

XVI Head Stand—*Sirshāsana*   Plates 27, 28, 29

A. Triangle Head Stand

1. Kneel, place the head on the floor, taking the weight on the upper part of the forehead at the hairline. Place the arms on the floor, elbows close to the knees, hands overlapping around the head in a firm grip. In this way a triangle is formed, with the weight at three points.

2. Straighten the legs, taking the weight on the forehead and toes. Walk up on the toes, bringing the knees close in to the chest. (See Plate 27)

3. Tuck the knees close to the chest, simultaneously giving a slight push off the floor with the toes. Fold the legs in jackknife

PLATE 27

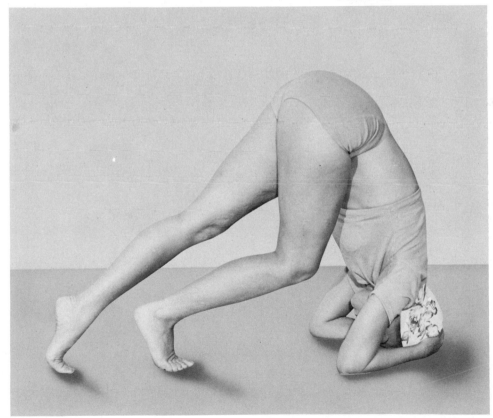

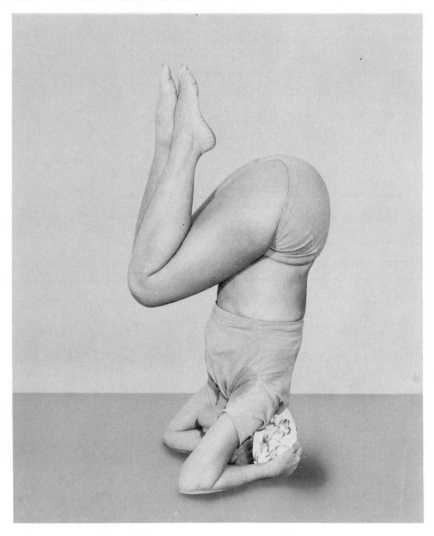

PLATE 28

position. Round the spine outward to a convex position. (See Plate 28)

4. Lift and straighten the legs slowly upward, gradually reversing the arch in the spine to a concave position. (See Plate 29)

5. Return slowly to first position in reverse sequence.

(See Variations, pages 143–144.   Plate 30)

Suggestions for Practice

Do not roll over to the top of the head. Keep the position on the forehead throughout.

Keep the maximum weight on the forearms, with as little as possible on the head.

Press the elbows into the floor, and do not allow them to spread apart from the triangle position.

PLATE 29

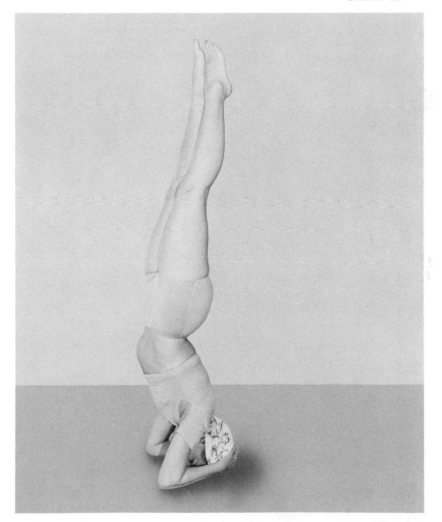

Tuck the knees into the chest as they are lifted and straightened.

Try not to jerk or kick the legs up into the air in learning to balance on the head. This has a tendency to throw the weight forward.

At the beginning it is a help to practice in a corner, or next to a wall. The support of the wall assists in maintaining the position, and in this way the benefits of the posture are gained even though it may not yet be possible to balance the body on the head and arms alone.

Another important help is to learn how to fall; then if the balance is lost there is no danger of hurting oneself. This can be done

PLATE 30

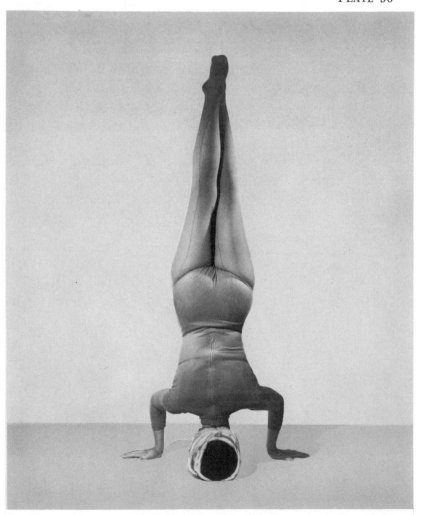

by practicing forward roll overs, or somersaults, with the knees closely tucked to the chest and the back well rounded. In this way fear of falling is overcome.

In coming down from a head stand, bend the knees in close to the chest, simultaneously reversing the arch in the spine. *The knees should be kept close to the chest until the feet touch the floor.* If the balance is lost in the opposite direction, bend the neck in reverse arch, or convex position, and roll over on the shoulders in a somersault. Relax while doing this, and the weight in falling will be accommodated naturally.

B. Tripod Head Stand   Plate 31

1. Kneel, place the head on the floor as described above, but this time with the hands palms down and turned outward in front of the knees, about as far apart as the width of the shoulders. The

PLATE 31

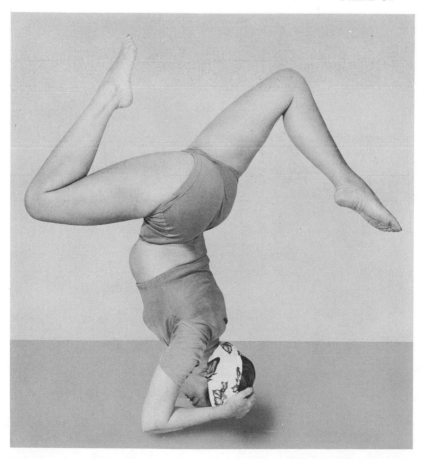

forearms should be kept at right angles to the floor, thus making a tripod with the head and hands.

2. Straighten the legs, taking the weight on the toes, hands, and head. Walk up on the toes, bringing the knees close to the chest.

3. Open the knees and place them on top of the bent elbows, simultaneously lifting the feet off the floor. Balance in this position for a few moments.

4. Lift and straighten the legs slowly upward, gradually reversing the arch in the spine to a concave position.

5. Return slowly to the first position, bringing the knees to the elbows and then placing the feet on the floor.

Do not allow the elbows to spread. Keep the forearms at right angles to the floor.

Note. See Lotus Head Stand, page 100.

MEDITATION POSTURES

The Meditation Postures have been designed to provide a firm base for keeping the spine in perfect alignment, so that the cir-

PLATE 32

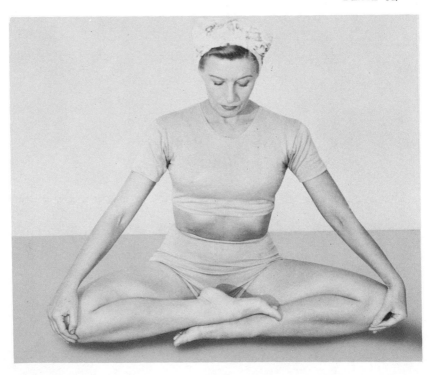

culation to the nervous system may be free and unimpeded. The spine is the switchboard of the body, closely connected with the brain, or main center. What the nervous system is to the body, the brain is to the mind, and the mind to the spirit. By holding the body still and erect, the mind is freed from its physical bondage and can be directed within.

XVII. Perfect Posture—*Siddhāsana*   Plate 32

1. Sit with the legs extended.

2. Bend the right knee and place the right heel at the perineum with the sole turned upward.

3. Bend the left knee and place the left heel over the right heel, or the top of left instep over the bottom of the right instep.

4. Hold the posture, maintaining the spine erect. The hands may be placed on the knees, palms down, or folded together with the palms up and resting on top of the feet. (See Plate 32)

PLATE 33

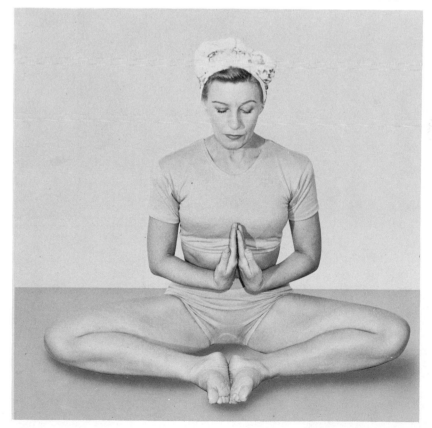

Suggestions for Practice

It is important to keep the knees on the floor, for this opens the hips and frees the entire pelvic region.

Do not slump or lean forward, but hold the spine erect and well elongated. This is imperative in order to obtain the greatest benefit from the breathing practices which are performed in this posture.

The three Locks may be taken in any of the Meditation Postures. Also in the breathing practices and the eye exercises.

(See Variations, pages 144–145.   Plate 33)

XVIII. Hidden Posture—*Guptāsana*   Plate 34

1. Sit with legs outstretched.

2. Bend the right knee and place the toes of the right foot in the left knee joint.

PLATE 34

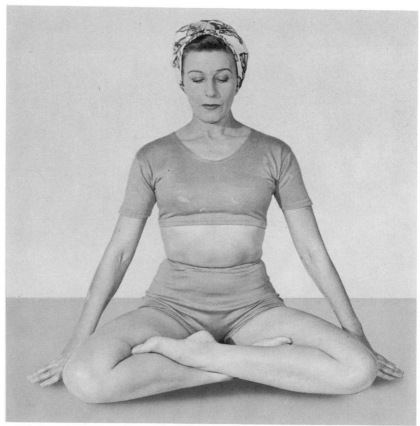

3. Bend the left knee, bring the left foot under the right knee joint. Thus the toes of both feet are hidden in the bend of the knees. Keep both knees on the floor. (See Plate 34)

4. Hold, maintaining the spine erect, hands on knees or feet.

This posture is useful in keeping the feet warm in cold weather. It is the least difficult of the Meditation Postures, and if practiced first, helps to make the others easier.

XIX. Lotus Posture—*Padmāsana*   Plate 35

1. Sit with the legs outstretched.

2. Bend the right knee and place the right foot on top of the left thigh at the groin, keeping the right knee down.

3. Bend the left knee and place the left foot on top of the right thigh at the groin, keeping the left knee down.

PLATE 35

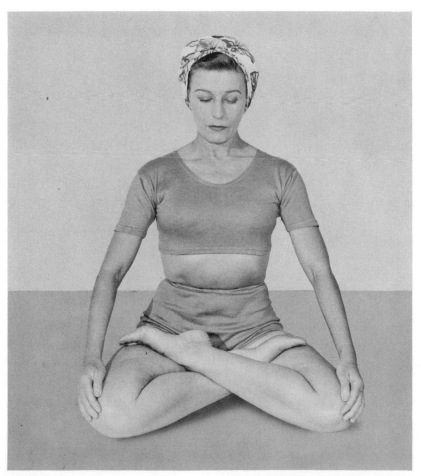

4. Hold, maintaining the spine erect, hands placed on the knees or feet. (See Plate 35)

Suggestions for Practice

Same as for the Perfect Posture.

An important preliminary for the Lotus Posture is the practice of the Leg-Folding exercises, as described in the Preparatory exercises (page 59). These should be done in both lying-down and sitting position until the knee joints are limbered up and the hips opened and stretched.

The Lotus Posture is the best of all positions in which to practice Meditation, since the lower limbs are locked together, thus providing a firm unshakable base.

In Meditation fixing the eyes is a further help to concentration (as in the practice called *Trātaka*).

The Eye Exercises are to be used in connection with the Meditation Postures as an aid to stilling the mind, and in focusing the attention within.

Eye Exercises—*Trātaka*

A1. Place a small bright object at eye level about five feet away.

2. Look at it steadily without blinking until tears begin to form.

3. Close eyes and hold image as long as possible.

B. Place lighted candle at eye level about five feet away. Look steadily without blinking until tears begin to form. Close eyes and hold the image as long as possible.

C1. Fix gaze on the tip of the nose.

2. Hold steadily without blinking.

D1. Fix gaze on imaginary point between the eyes.

2. Hold steadily without blinking.

Note. The eyes can be closed during this last exercise if preferred.

ADVANCED POSTURES

XX. Completed Lotus Posture—*Baddha Padmāsana*   Plate 36

1. Take Lotus Posture.

2. Cross the left arm behind the back and grasp the left toe.

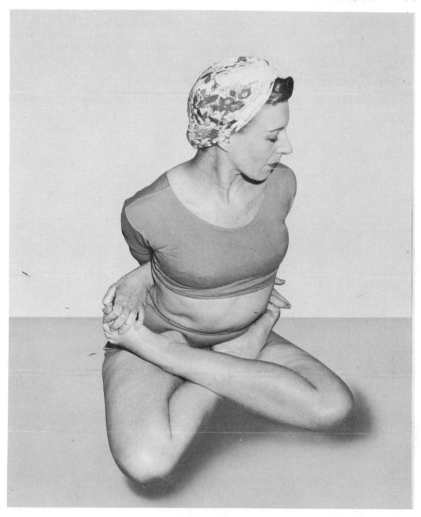

PLATE 36

3. Cross the right arm behind the back and grasp the right toe. (See Plate 36)

4. Hold.

This posture is used for the purpose of "locking off" the limbs of the body (both arms and legs) in order to create a greater pressure within the vital centers located in the trunk. It is used in advanced breathing practices, and is also beneficial as an exercise in itself for attaining a high degree of flexibility.

XXI. Lotus Head Stand—*Sirshāsana Padmāsana*   Plates 37,
38, 39

1. Take Lotus Posture.
2. Rock forward onto the knees.
3. Place head and hands in Tripod position. (Plate 37)
4. Slide knees (still in Lotus Posture) up to elbows. (See Plate
38)
5. Lift legs, keeping them in folded position, and raise them to
the Head Stand. (See Plate 39)

Suggestions for Practice

If preferred, the legs may be folded in the Lotus position *after*
the Head Stand has been assumed.

PLATE 37

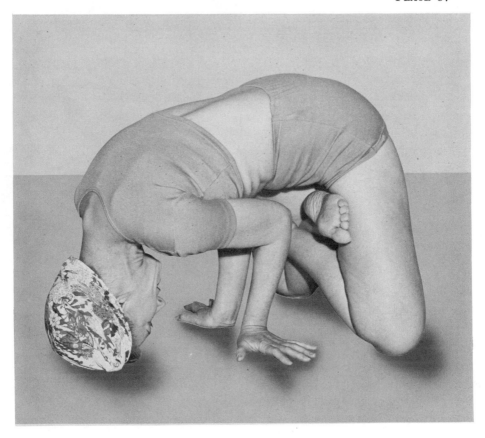

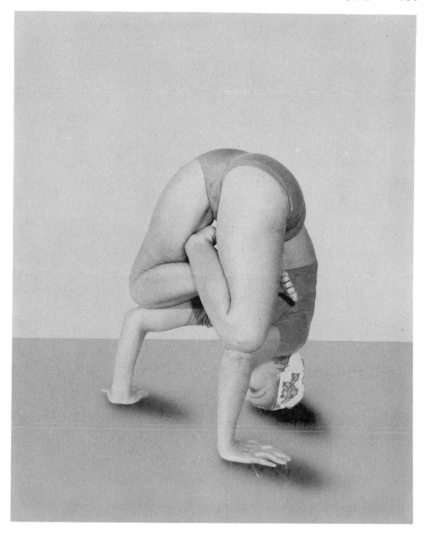

PLATE 38

First separately practice the Triangle and Tripod Head Stands and the Lotus Posture until they can be done easily; then the combination of the two in the Lotus Head Stand will not be found difficult. Both are splendid exercises for strengthening the spine and abdominal muscles.

The Lotus Head Stand can be taken in either the Tripod or Triangle positions.

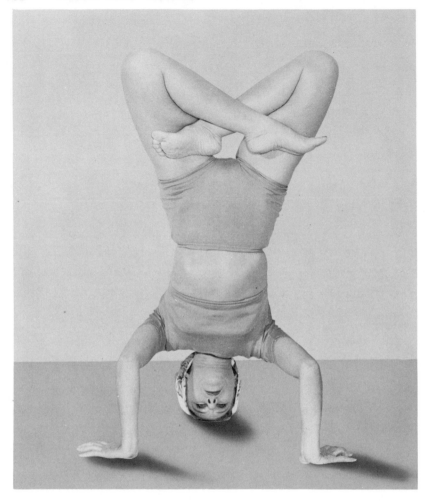

PLATE 39

XXII. Symbolical Posture—*Yoga Mudra*   Plate 40
   1. Take the Lotus Posture.
   2. Bend forward, keeping the hips on the ground, and touch the head to the floor.
   3. Stretch the arms forward and touch the hands to the floor.

Suggestions for Practice

If in the beginning it is difficult to touch the head to the floor, bend as far forward from the waist as possible and then return to

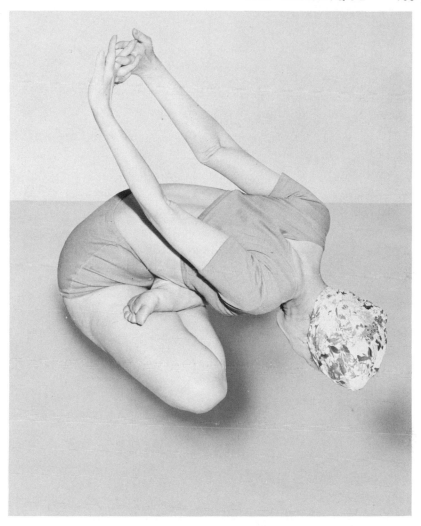

PLATE 40

the upright position. Repeat several times, bending forward a little more each time.

This posture may also be done with the arms extended behind the back, hands clasped (as in Plate 40).

When performed in this way it is especially beneficial to the shoulders, making them flexible, and also relieving nervous tension in the neck and at the base of the brain.

XXIII. Fish Posture—*Matsyāsana*   Plate 41

   1. Take Lotus Posture.

   2. Lie flat on the back, hands grasping the toes.

   3. Arch the neck and shoulders, rolling over onto the top of the head. (See Plate 41)

Suggestions for Practice

Do not lift the knees from the ground. Be sure to keep the hips flat.

This posture is especially good for stimulating the glands in the throat (thyroid and parathyroid) and also the vital organs that lie in the pelvic region—particularly the reproductive organs.

It can also be done with the arms folded over the head, keeping the neck and shoulders flat on the ground.

This is called the Fish Posture because when done in the water one can float without effort.

PLATE 41

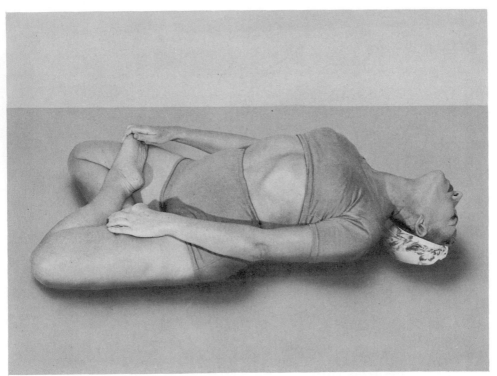

XXIV. Cock Posture—*Kukkutāsana*   Plate 42

1. Take the Lotus Posture.

2. Place the arms beside the hips, palms flat on the ground; press up, lifting the entire body several inches from the ground.

3. Hold, maintaining the balance on the hands. (See Plate 42)

Suggestions for Practice

If the Lotus Posture has not yet been perfected this exercise may be done in cross-legged position (sitting tailor fashion), then placing the hands beside the hips and lifting the body several inches off the floor. This is a good way to strengthen the muscles of abdomen, shoulders, back, and arms.

PLATE 42

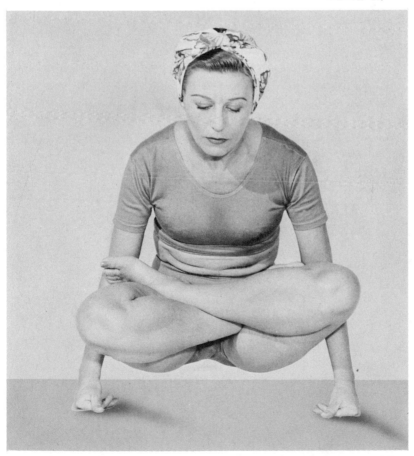

XXV. Peacock or Alligator Posture—*Mayurāsana*   Plate 43
    1. Take the Lotus Posture.
    2. Place the hands in front, palms down on the floor, about twelve inches apart with wrists facing in, fingers out. Roll up to the knees.
    3. Hook the elbows into the pelvic hollows above the hip bones, while remaining on the knees.
    4. Press up, lifting the knees as far as possible from the floor, balancing on the elbows and taking the entire weight on the hands. (Plate 43)

Note. This posture may also be performed without taking the Lotus Posture, instead keeping the legs extended.

Suggestions for Practice

It is important to shift the weight forward before attempting to lift the legs off the floor.

This posture brings pressure on the section of the large intestine located just above the hip bones: the ileocecal valve on the right side, and the sigmoid flexure on the left. Fecal matter has a tendency to lodge at these two points, and is sometimes difficult to eliminate even when the rest of the colon is clear. The Peacock Posture is helpful in draining residual water at these two points, when cleansing the colon as in *Basti,* page 128.

PLATE 43

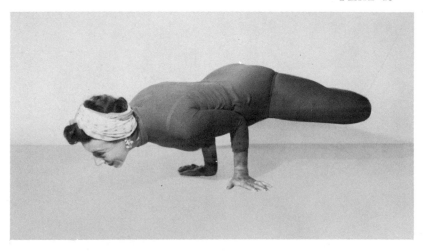

XXVI. Tree or Stork Posture—*Vrikṣāsana*   Plate 44

1. Stand erect.

2. Place the right foot in the left groin.

3. Bring the arms above the head and place the palms together, or cross the arms and clasp the elbows above the head. (See Plate 44)

4. Balance and hold. Then take the position balancing on the opposite leg.

PLATE 44

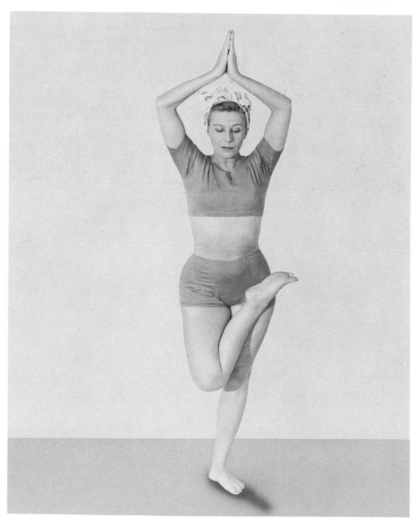

Suggestions for Practice

The purpose of this posture is to develop balance and steadiness. Therefore it should be held as long as possible without wavering. If the gaze is fixed on a point at eye level it is easier to maintain the balance.

BREATHING PRACTICES

The Yoga breathing practices are called *Pranayama,* from the Sanskrit *Prana*—breath—and *Ayama,* which means pause, or regulation. The aim of these practices is to control the breath in all its phases; inhalation *(Pūraka)*, retention *(Kumbhaka)*, and exhalation *(Rechaka)*. Before this control can be gained, here again as in all Yoga work, capacity must be first developed.

In the following exercises, whenever the breath is retained the three Locks are taken simultaneously, creating additional pressure, and thus causing greater absorption of oxygen (like putting the lid on a pressure cooker). When the breath is held there is a natural expansion of lungs, throat, and abdomen. The purpose of the Locks is to counteract the distention above and below, in throat and abdomen, thereby expanding the lung cavity to its utmost capacity. In this way lung cells normally unused are opened up and aerated, and as more surface is exposed, more oxygen will be absorbed.

Before beginning any of the following exercises, the lungs should first be completely emptied. This is best done by forcibly expelling the air through the mouth in short exhalations having the sound of "Ha." The residual air in the unused portions of the lungs is cleaned out and replaced with fresh air.

It is obvious that all stale air should be eliminated in order to benefit from holding the breath. If the breath is held without first cleansing the lungs, the carbon dioxide or waste product is retained, and this may cause dizziness and a feeling of pressure in the head.

The breathing practices may be done in any sitting position, though they are performed to best advantage in one of the Meditation Postures. The reasons for this are explained on page 94.

It is of course important to select a well-ventilated room for the breathing exercises. Best of all is to do them out of doors in some quiet, sheltered spot. *Pranayama* practiced in the mountains, at an altitude of 3,500 to 6,000 feet, brings special benefits.

PREPARATORY BREATHING EXERCISE

XXVII. Deep Cleansing Breath

1. Sit in one of the Meditation Postures, or any cross-legged or seated position, arms above the head.

2. Exhale forcibly through the *mouth* with "ha" sounds, while bending forward until the head and hands are touching the floor.

3. Inhale forcibly through the *nose,* raising the trunk to an upright position while the arms extend in a wide circle until the hands clasp at the back, palms down and pressing against the floor.

4. Retain the breath for a few seconds while holding the upright position with spine held straight.

The above constitutes one round. Repeat several times.

Suggestions for Practice

Be sure to keep the spine erect and the posture correct during the retention of the breath.

Do not let the hips leave the floor when bending forward, nor lift the knees up when pressing the palms down to the floor in back.

Do not thrust the head forward, but keep the chin in and the trunk and head well erect.

The *Deep Cleansing Breath* is especially valuable in ridding the lungs of residual air and in whipping up circulation. In bending forward, the air is squeezed out by means of the collapsed position of the lungs. In the upright position, with palms pressed on the floor at the back, the entire thoracic cavity is opened up and greatly expanded. The purpose in pressing the palms to the floor is to open the lungs by pushing the shoulders well back and down.

This exercise is an important preparation for the more advanced breathing practices.

BREATHING EXERCISES

XXVIII. Alternate or Nasal-Cleansing Breath—*Vāma Krama*

1. Close the right nostril with the right *thumb* pressed against

the right side of the nose. Inhale forcibly through the left nostril.

2. Close the left nostril by pressing the fingers of the right hand against the left side of the nose. Retain the breath for a few seconds.

3. Remove the right thumb from the right nostril and exhale forcibly keeping the left nostril closed.

4. Inhale forcibly through the right nostril.

5. Close the right nostril with the right thumb and retain the breath for a few seconds.

6. Remove the fingers from the left nostril and exhale forcibly through the left nostril, keeping the right nostril closed.

This constitutes one round. Repeat several rounds.

Suggestions for Practice

The breath should be kept flowing steadily in and out without interruption. Do not let it go between rounds.

Never allow yourself to get out of breath at any time. It is better to stop and rest until the breathing becomes normal before continuing another series of rounds.

Keep the spine erect and the posture correct throughout.

The Alternate Breath is of special benefit in cleaning out and opening up the nasal passages, and should be done at the beginning of the regular breathing practices. It has a calming effect on the entire system, and helps to focus the mind.

XXIX. Rhythmic Breath

1. Inhale through the nose   (4 or 16 counts).
2. Retain breath and take three Locks   (16 or 32 counts).
3. Release Locks, exhale through nose   (8 or 16 counts).

The above constitutes one round. Repeat several rounds.

Suggestions for Practice

In Rhythmic Breathing it is of paramount importance to keep the breath steadily flowing from one round to the next without interruption. Do not lose control of the breath at any time. Think of the ingoing and outgoing breath as "a silken cord that must not be broken."

It is better to augment the number of rounds than the number of counts (in the same ratio) within the round. As lung capacity and breath control are developed, the ratio can be doubled (i.e., from 4-16-8 to 8-32-16).

The individual pulse beat can be used to establish the tempo of one's personal rhythm.

The special Yoga breathing practices help to cleanse the post-nasal region of dust and dirt, thickened mucus in which germs collect causing sinus and middle-ear infections, colds, and many other diseases of the upper-respiratory tract. They also relieve congestion in the head and chronic catarrh.

XXX. Rhythmic Alternate Breath

Follow the same technique described in the Alternate Breath (XXVIII) at the same time controlling the inhalation, retention, and exhalation in the same ratio as the Rhythmic Breath.

1. Inhale through the left nostril   (4 or 8 counts).
2. Retain breath, both nostrils closed   (16 or 32 counts).
3. Exhale through right nostril, left closed   (8 or 16 counts).
4. Inhale through right nostril, left closed   (4 or 8 counts).
5. Retain breath, both nostrils closed   (16 or 32 counts).
6. Exhale through left nostril, right closed   (8 or 16 counts).

The above constitutes one round. Repeat several rounds.

XXXI. Bellows Breath—*Bhastrika*

1. Forcibly push out the air through the nose in a short, vigorous expulsion, simultaneously contracting the abdomen, diaphragm, and chest.

2. Release the contraction. The lungs will then automatically take in air.

3. Follow at once by another forcible expulsion.

4. Repeat a number of times in immediate succession. (For the beginner of average capacity, twenty times is enough. Later more can be added.)

5. On the final expulsion empty the lungs completely. Then inhale slowly, steadily, and forcibly through the nose to the full capacity of the lungs. Following this complete inhalation swallow, take the three Locks, and hold the breath as long as possible without strain.

6. After this retention, exhale very slowly and steadily; or preferably release the breath just a little at a time, taking in a small

amount of air after each exhalation until the lungs are empty. In this way the pressure is *gradually* released.

Suggestions for Practice

Keep the mouth closed and the throat open as if silently forming the syllable "ah." The nasal passages must remain free and open, with nostrils dilated.

Avoid any tension in the throat that might cause irritation, and any extraneous movements of the body, particularly of the facial muscles.

The expulsion of the breath should be deep and vigorous rather than quick and shallow. As power is developed, the speed of the contractions and expulsions may be increased. However, thoroughness should never be sacrificed for speed.

The practice of the Bellows Breath can be carried to a high state of proficiency. While at the beginning, a round should consist of a few breaths only, as strength develops the number and speed can be greatly increased. The usual number for the advanced student is 120 breaths a minute, constituting one round, and three rounds with retention between each round.

The Bellows Breath is the most important, exhilarating, and vital of all the Yoga breathing practices. It is, in fact, the supreme form of all exercise, and the most potent in its effect on the nervous system, and mind. It restores vitality and is a better antidepressant than any pill.

It is also best for eliminating the carbon dioxide that remains in the furthest recesses of the lungs and is untouched by ordinary breathing. The practice of the Bellows Breath accustoms the system to the habit of deeper breathing, and develops the capacity to take in more oxygen at all times. No other exercise so stimulates and increases the blood's capacity to absorb oxygen.

Bhastrika is sometimes called the *Runner's Breath,* for in this exercise the lungs, diaphragm, and abdominal muscles are, as in running, exerted to their utmost, while the body remains still in one position and physical force is not being expended to propel it through space.

The Bellows Breath is a reversal of the ordinary process of breathing, for here emphasis is on *exhalation* rather than on inhalation.

XXXII. Sighing Breath—*Ujjayi*

1. With the mouth closed and the throat (glottis) half open, draw the breath forcibly and evenly through the nose, making a sighing sound like gentle snoring.

2. Exhale forcibly and evenly, continuing the same sound.

This constitutes one round. Repeat several rounds.

Suggestions for Practice

Care should be taken not to close the glottis, but to keep it in a half-open position. If the throat is tight it may cause friction irritating to the mucous membranes.

The main purpose of this breathing practice is to massage and clean out the nasal passages, and to loosen the mucus at the back of the throat. It also has a calming effect on the entire nervous system.

XXXIII. Hissing, or Swan Breath—*Sītali* or *Hamsa*

1. Inhale forcibly through the nose until the lungs are completely filled.

2. With lips pressed against the teeth, expel the breath slowly and evenly, with a strong hissing sound.

The above constitutes one round. Repeat several rounds.

Suggestions for Practice

Keep the opening of the lips as small as possible, and try to increase the intensity of the sound by pressure of the breath.

The aim of the Hissing Breath is to gain control of the outgoing breath. As in the previous practice, it has a calming effect on the nervous system.

XXXIV. Droning Breath—*Brahmari*

1. Inhale forcibly through the nose until the lungs are completely filled.

2. With slightly parted lips and tongue pressed against the teeth, make a low humming sound, like the droning of bees, while expelling the breath steadily, slowly, and forcibly.

The above constitutes one round. Repeat several rounds.

Suggestions for Practice

Maintain as low a tone as possible while droning. Be sure that the sound is produced at the teeth and lips, and not in the nose. To determine whether this is being done correctly, hold the hand before the face and note whether air is coming from the mouth or the nose.

It is more important to increase the intensity of the vibration than to prolong the duration of the sound.

The main purpose of the Droning Breath is to gain control of the outgoing breath and to create a strong vibration through-out the entire nervous system.

This vibration is first felt in the head, then in the chest, and finally through the entire bodily structure. It acts like an inner massage, awakening every cell in the body, and is especially bene-ficial in stimulating the sensory organs. A noticeable improvement in hearing often follows after an extended period of this practice. Also the circulation to the sinuses and nasal passages is increased, helping to clear them of congestion.

Most important in the Droning Breath is the effect it has on the mind. By concentrating steadily on the droning sound, a state of intense quietude may be reached. For this reason it is helpful to practice *Brahmari* before Meditation.

The *Droning Breath* can also be done as follows:

1. Inhale forcibly through the nose until the lungs are com-pletely filled.

2. Place the thumbs in the ears, index fingers over the closed eyelids, middle fingers against the nostrils, fourth fingers against the upper lip, and fifth fingers against the lower lip.

3. Exhale with a low humming sound, as described in the above practice.

By stopping up the eyes, ears, nose, and mouth, all outside sounds and stimuli are cut off, and the inner vibration is greatly increased.

XXXV. Stretching Breath   Plate 45

1. Take a kneeling posture, with the head and shoulders touch-ing the floor, hands along the sides, palms up. Exhale completely. (See Plate 45)

2. Inhale slowly while rising to the knees, at the same time bringing the arms in a forward circle over the head. Clasp the hands together and stretch upward, raising the ribs high.

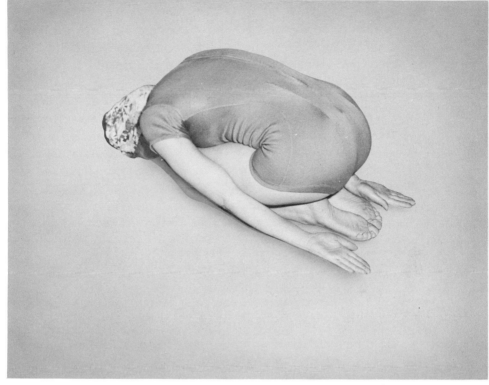

PLATE 45

3. Still retaining the breath, clasp the left wrist with the right hand and pull up and over to the right side, opening the ribs on the left.

4. Still retaining the breath, repeat the side stretch to the left, clasping the right wrist with the left hand.

5. Still retaining the breath, return to the central position with hands clasped over the head. Now unclasp the hands and make a big outward circle with the arms, bringing them down in back. The hands should be clasped with the palms down.

6. Exhale slowly, releasing the clasped hands and lifting the arms in a reverse inward circle over the head to the front. Then slowly return to the kneeling posture, bending forward and down to the first position, head on the floor. The exhalation should continue gradually and evenly throughout this sequence.

Relax and take several normal breaths before repeating.

Suggestions for Practice

First rehearse the above routine without holding the breath. Next go through the sequence with held breath but without the side stretches. When this can be done with ease and control, then do the complete exercise.

Do not bend forward at the hips when stretching to either side.

Be careful not to exhale in gasps, but control the outgoing breath in a steady flow. Or the breath can be released a little at a time, taking in a small amount of air after each exhalation.

The first position, kneeling with the head on the floor and arms at side, is beneficial to the spine and vital organs. It can be taken at any time for rest and relaxation.

The *Stretching Breath* is not strictly a Yoga breathing practice, but it has special value in reaching the outermost part of the lungs. By stretching during the retention of the breath, the air is forced into areas not ordinarily used.

The *Stretching Breath* should only be practiced after a degree of proficiency has been reached in the other breathing exercises.

ABDOMINAL EXERCISES

XXXVI. Hollow Tank—*Tadagi-Mudra*   Plate 46

1. Lie flat on the back with the knees up, feet on the floor.

2. Exhale vigorously and completely through the mouth.

3. With the breath held *out,* pull in the abdominal muscles. Maintain the contraction and draw up under the ribs as high as possible. Press the hands against the thighs to obtain extra resistance. (See Plate 46)

4. Hold as long as possible, then release the contraction and the air will automatically rush back into the lungs.

Take a few normal breaths and repeat several times.

Suggestions for Practice

Try to increase the intensity of the contraction, and especially the upward lift, as you hold the *Hollow Tank.*

On releasing the abdominal contraction there will be a natural inclination to gasp for air. Try to overcome this by taking in the breath a little at a time, keeping it under control at all times.

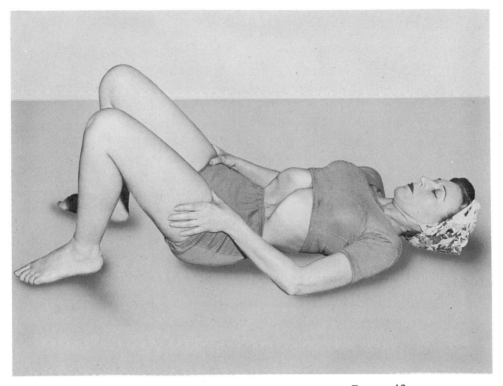

PLATE 46

The back and shoulders should remain pressed against the floor throughout the exercise.

The *Hollow Tank* is the *Solar-Plexus Lock* taken with the breath held out. It is especially good for lifting the muscles of the abdomen and diaphragm, and in opening the ribs; this in turn is a help to more efficient practice of all the breathing exercises. The strong inner suction lifts the vital organs, overcoming prolapsis, and creates a corresponding lift in the rectal muscles and lower pelvis. The suction or vacuum in the abdominal cavity presses against the nerve center at the Solar Plexus, stimulating it to greater activity, and generating heat.

The *Hollow Tank* can be used to great advantage in connection with other postures, such as the Spine Balance (page 84), the Back-Stretching Posture (page 71), etc.

(See Variations, pages 145–146.   Plates 8 and 22)

XXXVII. Pelvic Hollow Tank—*Vajroli-Mudra*   Plate 22–23
(Hollow Tank in Spine-Balance Position)
1. Lie flat on the back, arms at the side, palms down.
2. Exhale and take the *Hollow Tank*.
3. Simultaneously raise both the trunk and legs into a jackknife position, meanwhile sliding the palms forward along the floor and pressing down. (See Plate 22)
4. Hold as long as possible, then release the tension, inhale and return to the lying-down position.

The three following exercises are excellent preparations for the advanced practices of Power Whip (*Uddhiyana*) and Muscle Isolation (*Nauli*).

XXXVIII. Abdominal Lift   Plate 47
1. Lie on the back with the knees bent, feet on the floor. Rest the weight on the elbows, hands supporting the back.
2. Take the Hollow Tank, simultaneously exhaling. (Plate 47)
3. Release and expand the abdomen while inhaling.
This constitutes one round. Repeat several rounds in succession.

PLATE 47

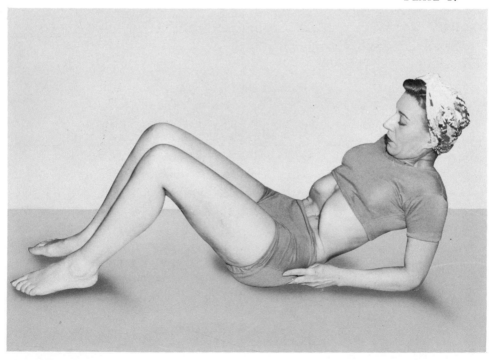

Suggestions for Practice

The Abdominal Lift must be done with a definite thrust both in and out, maintaining a rhythm that should be kept up without sacrificing thoroughness. It is helpful to do this to a count of three:

1. Pull in.
2. Lift up.
3. Let go.

The upward lift is the most important of the three.

This is not a breathing exercise, but the breath is important in maintaining the rhythm. With a little practice this rhythm becomes automatic.

The Abdominal Lift is especially useful in awakening intestinal activity, improving elimination and digestion, ridding the system of gas, and reducing excess abdominal fat.

XXXIX. Hammock Swing

1. Take same position as in the *Abdominal Lift*.
2. Exhale and do the *Hollow Tank*.
3. Push out the abdomen with a strong thrust to the *right,* at the same time inhaling.
4. Again exhale and take the *Hollow Tank*.
5. Push out the abdomen with a strong thrust to the *left,* at the same time inhaling.

This constitutes one round. Repeat several rounds.

Suggestions for Practice

Do not lift the hips from the floor at any time during this exercise.

The *Hammock Swing* brings the transverse abdominal muscles into play, and is a specific preliminary to *Nauli,* or *Muscle Isolation.*

XL. Cat Hump   Plate 48

1. Take position on the hands and knees.
2. Exhale, take the *Hollow Tank* and arch the back upward like a cat. (See Plate 48)
3. Release the contraction, inhale and thrust the abdomen downward, reversing the arch of the back from convex to concave.

This constitutes one round. Repeat several times.

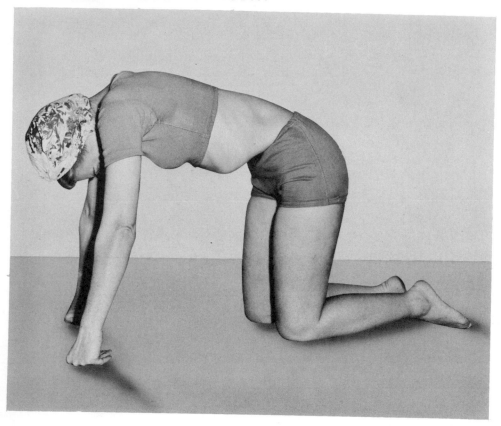

PLATE 48

Suggestions for Practice

Do not bend the elbows, but keep the arms straight.

Avoid rocking backward and forward on the hands and knees. Hold the position firmly fixed with the head down and the chin locked.

The *Cat Hump* gives a still higher lift to the abdomen than the previous exercises. It also exercises the spine and makes it flexible.

The *Hammock Swing* can also be done in the *Cat-Hump* position.

XLI. Abdominal Churn—*Lauliki*

1. Sit in cross-legged position, hands on the knees.
2. Exhale and take *Hollow Tank*.

3. Rotate the abdominal muscles to the right in circular motion.

4. Repeat several times, then inhale, again take the *Hollow Tank* and rotate to the left.

See Variation, page 146.

Suggestions for Practice

The hips must be kept on the floor throughout this exercise.

Grasp the knees firmly, keep the shoulders back, the spine straight, and the arms taut against resistance.

Do not bend forward at the waist. Pull against the knees with the arms and shoulders. Only the abdominal muscles should move; the rest of the body must be held firm.

The *Abdominal Churn* exercises all of the abdominal muscles, gives flexibility and tone to the entire abdominal section, acts like a churn on the intestines, and stimulates the bowels to proper elimination. (The Sanskrit *Lauliki* means churn.)

This exercise is a specific preparation for *Nauli*, or *Muscle Isolation*.

XLII. Power Whip—*Uddhiyana*   Plate 49

1. Stand with the legs apart, knees bent, hands pressing against the thighs.

2. Take the *Hollow Tank* with vigorous exhalation. (See Plate 49)

3. While holding the breath out, whip the abdomen in and up with a strong inner contraction. Then immediately release it.

4. *With the breath held out* repeat as many times as possible. Then inhale and take a few normal breaths.

This constitutes one round. Repeat several rounds.

Suggestions for Practice

Emphasis must be on the whiplike action of the contraction and lift, while the release in between is automatic and complete. Try to increase the power and intensity of the up and in, or "whip" stroke.

A rhythm should be established that can be maintained without overstrain.

The *Power Whip* may also be done in cross-legged position.

The practice of *Uddhiyana*, or the *Power Whip*, is one of the

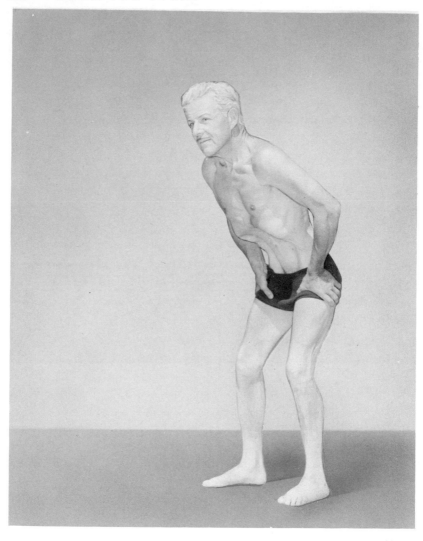

PLATE 49

most important of all Yoga exercises. A high standard of health could be maintained by this exercise alone.

The *Power Whip* stimulates all the vital functions of the body: the digestion, assimilation, circulation, nervous system, glands, and breathing. These results, however, can only be gained after intensity and strength have been developed, giving enough endurance to repeat the exercise many times.

It is essential to begin *slowly*. Daily practice with *gradual* increase of rounds is of special importance. At the start six to eight contractions on one exhalation will be enough, later increasing the number to twenty or more, as efficiency is developed.

XLIII. Muscle Isolation—*Nauli*   Plate 50

This exercise develops the two muscles on either side of the abdomen *(abdomini recti)* until they can be isolated, and is one of the most advanced of the Yoga practices.

PLATE 50

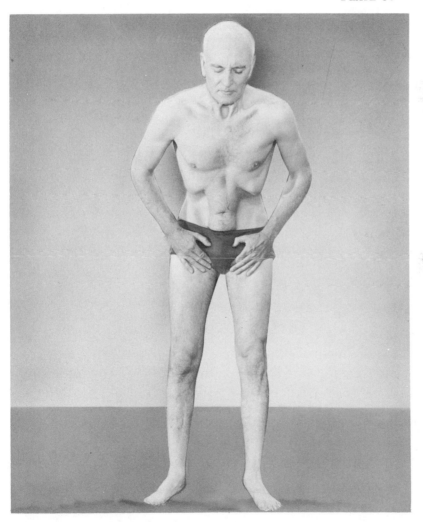

1. Stand with legs apart, knees bent, hands pressing against the thighs (same posture as in the *Power Whip*).

2. Take the *Hollow Tank* with vigorous exhalation.

3. While holding the breath *out,* press out the two abdominal muscles. (See Plate 50)

4. Repeat as many times as possible with the breath held out. Then inhale and take a few normal breaths.

This constitutes one round. Repeat several rounds.

When the above can be done (with both *abdomini* isolated) then practice with one at a time, isolating each in rotation as in the *Abdominal Churn.*

Suggestions for Practice

A certain amount of effort is naturally involved in this exercise, but care should be taken not to strain unduly. After the abdominal muscles have been well developed through perfecting the other exercises, no special strain should be necessary in isolating the *abdomini recti.*

In practicing *Nauli* it is helpful to stand in front of a mirror (if possible at a lower level). In this way the mental picture is connected with the muscular reaction.

Muscle Isolation is of great importance in developing suction in the abdominal cavity, in order to draw the muscles of the rectum up and in. This technique is used in performing *Basti,* a practice which cleanses the colon by creating a vacuum in the lower bowel and thereby sucking up water.

CLEANSING PRACTICES

In Hatha Yoga special Cleansing Practices (called *Dhautis*) are considered as necessary for the proper care of the body as brushing the teeth or bathing. No work on the theory and practice of this science would be complete without a description of the most fundamental of these *Dhautis.* Aside from maintaining the system in such condition that the greatest benefit from the work may be obtained, certain of the Cleansing Practices could be, on occasion, most valuable because of their simplicity and immediacy.

The exercises described below bring about a high standard of internal cleanliness to the mouth, nose, throat, stomach, and lower bowel.

XLIV. Nasal Cleansing or Elephant *Mudra—SitKrama* **or**
   Matangi Mudra

1. Take a large mouthful of water to which has been added a pinch of salt or some mild mouthwash.

2. Bend the head well forward over the basin.

3. Breathe in, close the glottis and push the water gently out through the nose while gradually exhaling. Repeat several times.

Suggestions for Practice

Do not *force* the water out through the nose, but hold the head well forward and down, and let the water flow through easily, without strain. The first few times a stinging sensation may be felt in the nose and a smarting in the eyes, but this is only a temporary symptom which will disappear as the passages are opened up and the mucous membranes become accustomed to the water. The general effects of this *Nasal Cleansing* practice are soothing and pleasant.

Nasal Cleansing may also be done by breathing in through the nostrils and at the same time gently snuffing water up the nose, then breathing out and expelling it through the mouth. Care should be taken not to force the water up, as it might then be pushed into the sinuses and ear passages.

Another means of *Nasal Cleansing* (called *Neti-Kriya*) is to insert a stiffened string (or the smallest-size catheter in place of the string) through one of the nostrils, bringing it out from the back of the throat through the mouth. Reverse this procedure through the other nostril. This practice should only be done under the personal supervision of a teacher.

XLV. Tongue Cleansing—*Jivha-Sodhana* **or** *Tongue Dhauti*

1. Extend the tongue as far forward as possible, keeping it flat.

2. Massage vigorously with three fingers at the base of the tongue.

Suggestions for Practice

To prevent gagging, take the *Hollow Tank* position while doing the *Tongue Cleansing* exercises, and keep the glottis well open.

Tongue Cleansing is a means of ridding the tongue and back of the throat of the mucus that drops down from the nose (post-nasal drip). It also dilates the glottis and by opening the throat plexus affects the nervous system.

Tongue Stretching (grasping the tongue by the fingers and pulling it—called milking) has much the same purpose as Tongue Cleansing. In addition it elongates the frenum, the membranous cord underneath the tongue that attaches it to the mouth. This is a necessary preparation for certain of the advanced breathing practices in which the tongue is turned backward and pressed against the soft palate to prevent any escape of air during prolonged retention of the breath.

Another exercise which stretches the frenum is called the *Lion Posture (Simāsana)*. This is performed in the following manner:

1. Kneel and sit on the feet.

2. Take the *Hollow Tank*.

3. Place the hands palms down on top of the thighs with fingers outstretched.

4. Extend the tongue outward and down, touching the chin if possible.

5. Open the eyes wide and fix the gaze without blinking. Try to bulge out the eyes in a fierce stare.

This posture should be held in complete tension. It is especially beneficial in preventing and alleviating sore throat.

XLVI. Stomach Cleansing—*Vamana-Dhauti*

1. Drink to full capacity six or more glasses of tepid water (a little salt may be added).

2. Open the throat by pressing the tongue down, taking the *Solar-Plexus Lock* and rolling the eyes upward.

3. Forcibly expel the water.

Suggestions for Practice

The *Solar-Plexus* Lock in conjunction with vigorous dilation of the throat muscles helps to overcome gagging or retching.

If the stomach is not completely emptied, drink more water and expel again.

The *Stomach-Cleansing* exercises eliminate excess mucus which causes overacidity and catarrhal conditions. A most important use of this practice is to induce immediate regurgitation if indigestible or poisoned food has been eaten. In cases of ptomaine poisoning the ability to empty the stomach rapidly may save life by preventing further assimilation of the poison into the system.

Cleaning out the stomach is also a splendid means of generally purifying the body. When used for this purpose the best time is before breakfast, when the stomach is entirely empty. Practice will bring ease and skill which at some later time may prove invaluable.

There are a number of other cleansing methods used in Hatha Yoga, such as *Dande-Dhauti*—cleansing the stomach by swallowing an oiled stomach tube, and *Vaso-Dhauti*—swallowing several yards of oiled gauze, but as these forms of Stomach Cleansing should only be practiced under the direction of a teacher, the detailed instructions are not included here.

THE YOGIC ENEMA

To apply with intelligence the Yoga principles of colon cleansing, it is first necessary to understand the structure and function of the alimentary tract, particularly of the large intestine or lower bowel.

The alimentary canal, from mouth to rectum, is twenty-seven to twenty-eight feet long. The large intestine, or colon, averages approximately five feet in length and about one and a half inches in diameter. The aim of the high enema is to reach the upper end of this large intestine where it joins the small intestine at the ileocecal valve. This valve is a one-way opening, preventing fecal matter from the colon backing up into the small intestine. Here too is located the appendix, called from its shape *vermiform*, or "wormlike," a sac usually three to four inches in length. Inflammation of the appendix is often the result of chronic constipation.

By the time food reaches the large intestine it has chiefly become waste substance, most of the digestive properties having been absorbed while in the small intestine. If this waste matter is allowed to remain in the colon beyond its normal period, an absorption of toxic by-products takes place. Hence the dangers of constipation.

The old-fashioned attitude toward the enema is rapidly changing. It is no longer looked upon as a major operation, only to be used in times of sickness, for today colon cleansing is advocated by most of the modern health, beauty, and reducing courses.

The Yoga enema, using the principles of the original colon cleansing called *Basti* (see below), is far more efficacious than the ordinary kind. In this practice the lower intestine is cleaned out by means of water retained in the lower bowel while doing certain of the abdominal exercises and postures. These exercises increase the normal peristaltic action—automatic, wavelike muscular contractions within the lining of the intestines—and cause the water to flush through every part of the colon. In this way a speedy and complete emptying of the lower intestine is brought about.

Cleansing out the colon is an immediate specific for counteracting depression, fatigue, nerve tension, and the effects of dissipation. Following a thorough internal housecleaning a delightful sense of well-being is felt, and a fresh and healthful attitude toward life is restored.

First a "low" enema should be taken. The purpose of this is to empty the lower section of the bowel (the sigmoid flexure) and to free the exit of fecal matter or gas, so that the high enema may be taken without encountering obstruction or the discomfort caused by gas.

The low enema may be advantageously used whenever fecal matter is present in the rectal vault, and has not been normally evacuated. This lower section of the colon should always be free of waste matter, particularly before retiring at night. If at any time there is difficulty in evacuating, it is better to take a low enema than to strain. This will dissolve the hardened feces, making an easier and more complete movement possible.

XLVII. Colon Cleansing—*Basti*

1. In squatting position take a low enema, about a pint of water at tepid or blood temperature. The container or enema bag should be placed at about shoulder height, and a longer tip than usual is advisable. (A hard rubber vaginal tip may be used, with a little lubricant to facilitate insertion.)

Do not retain the water, but eliminate it at once.

2. Refill the container with two quarts of warm (not hot) water. A teaspoon each of salt and soda may be added, to counteract acidity.

3. Take the knee-chest position, contracting the abdomen as in the *Hollow Tank* (page 116) with breath held out. Let the water flow in as slowly as possible, then relax, take a normal breath and

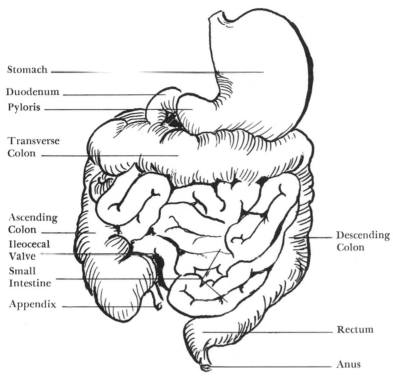

Stomach

Duodenum

Pyloris

Transverse
Colon

Ascending
Colon

Ileocecal
Valve

Small
Intestine

Appendix

Descending
Colon

Rectum

Anus

repeat, thus drawing the water in by suction and making the rectal and abdominal muscles work in cooperation.

4. Retain the water a few minutes, and do abdominal exercises before expelling.

5. Expel the water in small amounts, but forcibly; then shut off. This is an important means of strengthening the rectal muscles and bringing them under control.

Suggestions for Practice

Do not eliminate the water until the full two quarts has been taken into the colon. Should elimination be imperative before the full amount has been taken in, what has been lost should be replaced by additional water.

Avoid if possible getting into an upright position during the intake, as it will make retention more difficult.

Never strain. Dilate and contract the rectal muscles with each elimination.

A low stool twelve to fifteen inches high on which to place the feet during elimination will be found helpful. In this way a squatting position can be maintained. This is man's natural position for evacuation.

It is important that *all* of the water should be eliminated, as fecal matter in a liquid condition is easily absorbed. The Head Stand and Peacock Posture are helpful in accomplishing a thorough emptying.

When all of the liquid has been expelled, it is a good idea to sip a glass of hot water together with air swallowing (see following description). This will help to wash down anything that might still remain in the colon. As a final aid to relaxation, a rectal dilator inserted for five or ten minutes is helpful.

XLVIII. Air Cleansing—*Vatasara Dhauti*

One of the *Dhautis,* or inner purifications, in the Yoga work, is swallowing air. In this practice air is taken directly into the stomach, passes through the intestinal tract, and out through the rectum. It also increases peristaltic action. Sodium bicarbonate works on a like principle, producing extra gas to relieve what is already there. By swallowing air the same results may be obtained.

For the beginner it is helpful to take air and water together. Sip the water (preferably hot) while at the same time sucking in air, then dilate the muscles of the throat, open as in a yawn and swallow hard. The glottis should be closed so the water and air go into the stomach and not into the lungs.

In Yoga practice there are several methods of air swallowing. The most important of these are the *Crow-Bill Mudra (Vatasara-Dhauti)* and *Plavini-Mudra.*

Crow-Bill Mudra. Extend the lips and suck in large gulps of air, swallowing it directly into the stomach.

Plavini-Mudra. Same as above, at the same time taking the *Hollow-Tank* posture and pressing down the tongue with the fingers, opening the throat and swallowing large quantities of air.

Air swallowing is only to be practiced when the system has been well cleaned out. Otherwise feces obstructing the intestines may cause gas. If any discomfort is felt, lie on the left side and bring the right knee to the chest. Or take the knee-chest position. The Head Stand and Peacock Posture also help to relieve gas pressure.

SUPPLEMENTARY EXERCISES

A few additional exercises for the neck and shoulders are here included. They are helpful in offsetting the strains and occupational tensions so prevalent in modern living.

One of the most common of these is caused by leaning over a desk or machine, driving a car, playing a musical instrument, bending over housework, etc. In all these activities the muscles of the neck, hands, and shoulders are involved, and much less fatigue would be felt if occasionally during the day a few moments were given to relaxing these special muscle groups.

The following exercises are designed to untie muscular knots and nerve impingements in the above-mentioned regions. The neck exercises relieve this tension; they also help to keep down superfluous flesh at the back of the neck (sometimes called a dowager's hump) and they send a fresh flow of blood to the fifth cervical nerve at the base of the skull. This nerve affects the brain. Also special senses such as sight and hearing are stimulated by the neck exercises.

The Shoulder Shrugs strengthen the muscles that lift the breasts, and help to prevent their sagging and drooping.

Neck Exercises
   A1. Sit erect, lock chin.
     2. Jerk head over right shoulder, forcing chin out.
     3. Drop head backward, chin up.
     4. Jerk head over left shoulder, chin out.
     5. Relax and drop head forward, chin touching chest.
   B1. Rotate head to right, against resistance.
     2. Rotate head in opposite direction, against resistance.
     3. Rotate head relaxed.
   C1. Sit erect, drop head forward.
     2. Place fingers at base of skull and massage.
     3. Force head backward against pressure of fingers.
     4. Relax and drop head forward.
   D1. Take Cat-Hump position (XL).
     2. Drop head forward and shake vigorously.
     3. Lift head and force backward.
     4. Relax and drop head forward.

Shoulder Shrugs

    1. Shrug left shoulder as high as possible. Repeat several times.

    2. Shrug right shoulder in same manner.

    3. Shrug both shoulders together.

VARIATIONS

A number of variations to be used in connection with the Postures are here included. In the original Yoga work the Postures are intended to be held for some time. This, however, requires a high degree of flexibility. The following exercises help to give that extra flexibility necessary for maintaining the Postures without discomfort.

Endless variations can be devised. The Postures are a framework on which these may be built. Each student is free to use his own imagination in adapting the Yoga principles and in working out further elaborations. If this is done, the practice becomes creative and progressive, rather than static and perfunctory.

Variations of Half Posture (I)—*Virāsana*   Pages 63–64

    1. Sit in Half Posture—left leg folded against thigh, right leg bent with foot in opposite groin. (Plate 1)

    2. Grasp the inside of the right heel with the right hand, palm downward, and extend the leg forward and up until both the knee and the arm are straight. Repeat this extension several times, each time returning the foot to the groin.

    3. Again extend the leg forward and up. This time lower it to the floor in slow extension, maintaining the grasp on the heel and keeping the body erect.

    4. Repeat the above sequence with the left leg, right leg folded against the thigh.

Variations of "V" Posture (II)   Pages 64–66

A

    1. From "V" Posture (kneeling, with legs crossed) bend forward on the right knee.

    2. Gradually transfer the weight to the left foot and rise to an upright position, making a half turn to the right. When the half turn is completed, you should be standing upright with the weight equally balanced on both feet, and the feet about twelve inches apart.

3. Continue turning right by pivoting on the balls of the feet. Gradually bend the knees and transfer the weight to the left leg until the left knee touches the floor.

4. Return to "V" Posture, finishing the turn with the right knee on top of the left. Repeat the whole turn in the opposite direction.

This is sometimes called the V Twist or Corkscrew Turn.

B

The Low Corkscrew Turn.

From the "V" Posture make the corkscrew turn as in A without rising to upright position. Keep as close to the floor as possible in squatting position while making the pivot, with the weight balanced well forward over the balls of the feet. The arms may be clasped over the head or at the chest.

Suggestions for Practice

Control the balance carefully when returning to the "V" Posture after completing the pivot turn. This is a splendid exercise for improving the balance and for strengthening the ankles and insteps.

Variations of Frog Posture (III)   Pages 67–68

A

1. Take Frog Posture (sitting on heels in squatting position).

2. Balance on the balls of the feet and roll slowly forward on the toes until the knees touch the floor.

3. Roll back on the toes, lifting the knees from the floor, and return to the squatting position (Frog Posture).

Note. The hips should touch the heels throughout, and the pull should be strongly felt in the toes and insteps. Do not let the knees hit the floor with a bang, but lower them gradually.

B

1. Take Frog Posture (squatting position).

2. Rise slowly to upright position on the toes.

3. Remain standing, knees straight, and rock from the toes to the heels, raising toes from the floor and turning them up.

4. Remain standing and rock forward again to the toes. Repeat several times.

5. Slowly bend the knees and return to the Frog Posture.

See *Suggestions for Practice* for Frog Posture, pages 67–68.

Variation of Spine Twist (V)   Pages 69–70

1. Sit with the legs extended in front. Place the left foot flat on the floor to the right side of the right thigh. Bring the left knee up as close to the chest as possible.

2. *Keep the right leg extended.*

3. Twist the waist to the left until the back of the right elbow can be hooked over against the left arm.

4. Stretch and hold. Repeat opposite way.

This is sometimes called the Half-Twist Posture. It is not quite as difficult as the complete Spine Twist, and is therefore easier for the beginner.

Very beneficial results are obtained from this posture because of the stretch and pull which is given to the whole length of the spine, and to the shoulders and waistline as well.

Variations of the Back-Stretching Posture (VI)   Pages 71–74

A

1. Sit with the legs extended in front.

2. Stretch the arms over the head, and swing forward to touch the toes without bending the knees. (See Plate 8)

3. Return to erect position and forcibly bend the arms at the elbows. Bring the elbows close to the sides and to the back, throwing the chest open.

4. Repeat several times.

B

The above exercise can also be done as a breathing practice:

1. Exhale on the forward swing, grasping the toes.

2. Inhale and bend the elbows as the body is straightened.

3. Hold the inhalation and stretch the arms over the head.

4. Return to the first position and repeat.

C

1. Sit with the legs extended, knees straight.

2. Bend forward and grasp the toes.

3. Pull the heels off the floor, keeping the knees straight.

4. Hold the posture and take the three Locks.

Note. By lifting the heels off the floor, if only for an inch, an additional pull is given to the muscles in the back of the legs, the hamstrings. These muscles are usually somewhat shortened, especially in women who habitually wear high heels.

D

(Padhahastāsana)

1. Stand erect, feet together.
2. Bend forward from the waist, clasping the hands behind the ankles without bending the knees.
3. Touch the head to the knees, and chest to thighs. (See Plate 10)
4. Hold the posture and take the three Locks.

Note. This posture may be done with the legs separated (about two feet apart), swinging the head through the legs.

E

1. Sit with the legs extended in front.
2. Bend forward and grasp the toes.
3. Raise the legs off the floor as far as possible, maintaining the grasp on the toes.
4. Hold by balancing on the coccyx (end of the spine).

For *Suggestions for Practice* see Back-Stretching Posture, pages 71–74.

Variations for Pelvic Posture (VIII)   Pages 75–77

A

1. Take the Pelvic Posture with the knees close together, toes touching in back under the hips.
2. Turn the insteps down, the tops of the arches on the floor.
3. Separate and open the heels as far as possible, so that the arches of the feet form a cup, or basket, for the hips to sit in. The hips should be firmly touching the floor.

This posture is called *Swastikāsana.*

B

1. From the Pelvic Posture rise slowly to the knees, holding the spine straight and the hips pressing forward and under.
2. Return slowly to the Pelvic Posture without bending at the waist.
3. Repeat several times.

C

1. Same exercise as B, but this time lean back from the hips, to create a greater pull. Keep the spine straight and each time gradually increase the backward leaning angle.

2. Repeat several times.

D

1. Take the Pelvic Posture and grasp the insteps (or ankles) and rise to the knees while retaining the grasp of the feet.

2. Strongly arch the spine and open the shoulders, bending the head back between the shoulders. (See Plate 13)

3. Return to the Pelvic Posture by bending at the waist and hips, still retaining the grasp of the feet. Repeat.

Note. If it is too difficult at first to hold the feet, then place the hands palms down on the floor near the feet when doing the exercise.

E

1. From the Pelvic Posture rise to the knees, arch the back as much as possible and slowly lean back from the knees until the head touches the floor. (See Plate 14)

2. Return to the knees, keeping the back bent. The arms may be extended forward, hands placed on top of thighs, palms down or crossed at chest, or overhead.

Note. If this exercise is difficult in the beginning, try leaning back only a little, gradually increasing the arch.

F

1. From the Pelvic Posture shift the weight to the left leg, sitting on the left foot.

2. Bring the right knee to the chest, placing ball of right foot on the floor, and shifting the weight to it.

3. Bring the left knee to the chest, placing ball of left foot on the floor. The weight should now be balanced on both feet, as in the Frog Posture.

4. Return to the Pelvic Posture in reverse order, shifting the weight first to the ball of the right foot, then weight on right knee, sitting on the right foot. Next place the left knee on the floor, taking the weight on it, and sit between the legs in the Pelvic Posture.

Note. By placing the balls of the feet slightly ahead each time, this exercise can be done progressing forward. It is called the Duck Waddle. There is no better exercise for reducing the hips.

G

1. From the Pelvic Posture place the hands on the floor between the thighs, palms down, fingers outward, inside of wrists together. Lean forward with the weight on the hands.

2. Keep the weight on the hands, without changing their position. With a slight spring, lift the legs from the floor, bringing the knees to the chest as in the Frog Posture.

3. With another spring, lift the legs and return to the Pelvic Posture, keeping the weight on the hands until the hips touch the floor.

Note. This exercise also is splendid for hip reducing and for attaining lightness and flexibility in the legs. Speed should gradually be developed in performing this exercise.

H

1. From the Pelvic Posture jump to the Frog Posture, as in G2.

2. Keeping the weight on the hands, with a slight spring lift both legs off the floor and kick straight back. The weight should be equally balanced on the hands and toes, without touching the rest of the body to the floor. Keep the spine firm and in a semi-arch. Do not let the body sag in the middle.

3. With a slight spring, lift the legs and return to the Frog Posture in reverse sequence.

4. From the Frog Posture return to the Pelvic Posture, as in G3, completing the sequence.

Suggestions for Practice

In the last two sequences it is important to keep the weight on the hands to facilitate the legs in springing.

Variations of Supine-Pelvic Posture (IX)   Pages 78–80

A

1. Take the Supine Pelvic Posture and raise the knees, keeping the feet on the floor.

2. Grasp the ankles, arch the back and raise the hips, back, and shoulders from the floor. Keep the head on the floor and roll back to the top of the head, or forehead, if possible.

3. Maintain the hold of the ankles and raise and lower the trunk several times in succession, rolling back to the top of the head each time.

This posture is sometimes called The Wrestler's Bridge. It is very beneficial in keeping the neck, throat, and chin muscles firm.

B

1. Take the Supine-Pelvic Posture and raise the knees, keeping soles of feet on the floor, close to the sides of the hips.

2. Place hands, palms down, at the side of the shoulders, elbows bent at right angles to the floor. (Plate 16)

3. Raise shoulders, back, and hips from the floor, and arch upward by pushing simultaneously with the hands and feet. The elbows should straighten as you rise into the arch, and the knees should be partially straight. If possible lift the heels from the floor, taking the weight on the balls of the feet. Let the head drop back between the shoulders. (See Plate 17)

4. Lower the body to the floor by bending the elbows and knees and flattening out the back, returning to the Supine-Pelvic Posture.

This posture is sometimes called the Crab, or Circle (Chakrāsana).

C

1. Take the Crab Posture and extend one leg straight up or bent at right angles. (See Plate 18)

2. Repeat with opposite leg extended.

D

1. Stand with the feet about twelve inches apart. Raise the arms straight over the head, hands bent back at the wrists, palms up.

2. Slowly bend backward, making a complete arch in the spine from hips to head. In bending back, keep the weight forward over the feet by slightly bending the knees. Force the hips forward and open, drop the head back between the shoulders and keep bending until the hands touch the floor. The weight should be on the palms and balls of the feet, heels lifted from the floor.

3. Return to upright position, rocking forward, pushing up with the hands and taking all the weight on the feet. Straighten the knees when about halfway up.

Note. This exercise is the same as B, taking it from a standing instead of a lying-down position. (Supine Pelvic)

Suggestions for Practice

Keep the arms straight when arching the back to the floor. If the elbows are bent the head may hit the floor.

LYING-DOWN POSTURES

Variations of Cobra Posture (X)   Pages 80–81

A

1. Take the Cobra Posture.
2. Swing the upper body to the right from the waist in as big a circle as possible, bending to the right side and arching backward.
3. Next, bend to the left and then forward, with the chest touching the floor. The hands should remain pressed against the floor without changing their position. At the same time the head makes a smaller circle, following the movements of the trunk. The chin should be extended forward throughout.
4. Repeat, circling to the left.

B

1. Take the Cobra Posture.
2. Walk around on the hands to the right side of the body, twisting at the waist. The shoulders should be kept parallel and the head turned to the right, looking over the right shoulder.
3. Repeat to the left.

C

1. Take the Cobra Posture.
2. Press back into the Kneeling Posture, keeping the chest to the floor.
3. Sit on the feet, shoulders to knees, and head touching the floor.
4. Return to Cobra Posture, keeping the chest close to the floor throughout.

See *Suggestions for Practice* for Cobra Posture.

Variations of Locust Posture (XI)   Page 82

A

1. Take the Locust Posture with the hands clasped behind the head, instead of at the sides.

2. Press the legs up from the hips, and at the same time force the head back against the hands.

3. Hold.

B

1. Take the Locust Posture with arms outstretched up and forward, about three feet apart.

2. Roll over to the left on the hips to the Spine-Balance Posture (Variation A) maintaining the arms outstretched.

3. Roll back to the first position (Locust Posture with arms outstretched).

4. Repeat, rolling to the opposite direction.

Note. In the first position (B), the front of the hips only are touching, and in the second the balance is on the end of the spine, or coccyx. The legs and arms must be well off the floor, and the shoulders as well.

Variations of Bow Posture (XII)   Page 83

A

1. Take the Bow Posture.

2. Rock back and forth on the abdomen. This is done by dipping the head forward, and at the same time pressing the feet against the hands.

B

1. Lie on the abdomen.

2. Cross the right leg over the left at ankles. Grasp the left foot with the right hand, and the right with the left. Arch the back strongly.

3. Hold, or rock back and forth as in A.

Variations of Spine-Balance Posture (XIII)   Pages 84–85

A

1. Lie flat on the back.

2. Raise the upper body and the legs only a little from the floor. Balance on the end of the spine, or coccyx. (See Plate 23)

3. Hold until vibration is strongly felt in the abdomen and back, and there is a sensation of heat.

B

1. Take the posture as in A2. (Low Spine Balance)

2. Tuck the knees sharply to the chest in jackknife position, clasping them tightly, or with arms folded across the chest.

3. Return to first position. Repeat several times.

C

1. Take Low Spine-Balance position.

2. Open and close the legs sharply, like scissors, maintaining the Spine Balance throughout. Keep the legs as far off the floor as possible.

D

1. Take Low Spine-Balance position.

2. Pedal with the legs as if treading water, or bicycling.

E

1. Take Low Spine-Balance position.

2. Roll to the right hip, and bring the knees up in jackknife position, the feet touching the hips.

3. Extend the legs and roll onto the opposite hip, repeating the jackknife position.

4. Return to first position and repeat in opposite direction.

Note. These variations of the Spine-Balance Posture are especially good for reducing the hips and abdomen.

Variations of Shoulder Stand (XIV)   Pages 85–87

A

1. Take the Shoulder Stand, but this time keep the hands on the floor instead of at the small of the back.

B

1. Take the Shoulder Stand, placing the hands over the head, either extended or clasping the elbows.

C

1. Take the Shoulder Stand.

2. Bend the knees in jackknife position to the right shoulder.

3. Straighten the knees and bend them over the left shoulder.

4. Return to first position—legs extended upward.

D

1. Take the Shoulder Stand.

2. Tense the leg muscles, then relax and shake them.

E

1. Take the Shoulder Stand.
2. Open and close the legs like scissors.

F

1. Take the Shoulder Stand.
2. Pedal with the legs as if riding a bicycle.

See *Suggestions for Practice* for Shoulder Stand (pages 85–87).

Variations of Plough Posture (XV)   Pages 87–88

A

1. Take the Plough Posture.
2. Place the arms over the head, clasping the elbows.
3. Push the toes further over the head, as a plough making furrows.
4. Continue "ploughing."

B

1. Take the Plough Posture.
2. Bend the knees and bring to the shoulders, keeping the lower legs on the floor. (Plate 26)

C

1. Take the Shoulder Stand.
2. Bring the legs alternately over the head, touching the toes to the floor.

D

1. Take the Shoulder Stand.
2. Lower the legs very slowly to the Plough Posture.
3. Return the legs slowly to the Shoulder Stand. This is done by gradually rolling forward and backward on the spine.

E

1. Take the Shoulder Stand.
2. Swing the right leg over the left shoulder and touch the toe to the floor.
3. Swing the left leg over the right shoulder and touch the toe to the floor.

F

1. Take the Shoulder Stand.
2. Swing both the legs over the right shoulder, touching the toes to the floor.
3. Bring both the legs over the left shoulder, again touching the floor with the toes.

G

1. Take the Plough Posture.

2. Make a complete circle with both legs from the hips, touching the floor over the head, at sides and in front.

3. Repeat in opposite direction.

See *Suggestions for Practice* for Plough Posture.

Variations of Head Stand (XVI)   Pages 89–94

A. Swastika

1. From a standing position lunge forward on the right leg, dropping to the left knee.

2. Rock forward to the right knee. The weight of the trunk should be well forward over the right knee.

3. Place the arms and head on the floor in triangle position.

4. Swing the left leg over the head, with knee bent, simultaneously taking the weight on head and arms.

5. Lift the right leg overhead, knee bent. (Plate 31) The knees bent and separated in a straight line form the Swastika position.

In coming down from the Swastika Head Stand bring the right knee close to the chest, until the foot touches the floor. The left leg should swing in a big arch to the floor, returning to the second position indicated above. Then rock back onto the left knee and stand.

Suggestions for Practice

Keep the spine well arched, in concave position, throughout the exercise.

The knees should be separated as far as possible at all times.

Note. While maintaining the Swastika Head Stand the position of the legs may be changed, bringing the left knee back and the right knee forward, then returning to the floor by drawing the left knee to the chest.

B. Willow Tree

1. Take the Triangle Head Stand.

2. Open the legs and bend the knees back over the head. Arch the spine in concave position.

Suggestions for Practice

Keep the elbows firmly pressed into the floor. This will avoid the tendency to go over backward.

C. Jackknife

1. Take the Willow-Tree Head Stand.

2. Tuck the knees to the chest with a definite thrust, at the same time reversing the arch in the spine from a concave to a convex position. The feet should not touch the floor when in the Jackknife position.

3. Return to the Willow-Tree position.

Suggestions for Practice

Open the hips well when in the Willow-Tree position.

Be sure to make a full reversal of the arch in the spine when changing from the Jackknife position to the Willow Tree.

Note. This is a splendid exercise, when repeated several times, for limbering up the spine, hips and torso.

D. Splits in Head Stand

1. Take the Triangle Head Stand.

2. Open and close the legs like scissors (front split).

3. Open and close the legs to the side (side split).

4. Bicycle with the legs, still remaining in Head Stand.

E. Pull-up Head Stand

1. Lie flat on the abdomen, arms in Triangle position.

2. Pull up into the Head Stand, keeping the legs straight.

3. Come down, slowly lowering the legs and keeping them straight until the feet touch the floor. Then slide the feet back along the floor, returning to the first position (flat on abdomen).

Variations of Perfect Posture (XVII)   Pages 95–96

A

1. From the Perfect Posture rise to the knees, lifting the hips off the floor and pressing them forward over the feet.

2. Open the legs backward from the knees (as in Kneeling Posture) and sit in the Pelvic Posture.

3. Return, rising to the knees and folding the feet as in the first position.

4. Sit in back of the feet, in Perfect Posture.

Suggestions for Practice

In rising to the knees keep the hips open and forward.

Do not lean forward from the waist at any time during this exercise. Try to hold the body as erect as possible.

Move very gradually from one position into the next, especially when returning to a sitting position. Do not lose control and "let go."

Note. This exercise is very good for the hips, helping to keep down their weight, and making them flexible. In going from the Perfect Posture to the Pelvic Posture the hip joints make a complete turn in their sockets.

B

1. Bring the soles of the feet together, turning them up if possible. Keep the knees flat on the floor.

2. Place the backs of the hands together and bring them to the chest. (Plate 33)

Variations of the Hollow Tank (XXXVI)   Pages 116–117

The following variations of the abdominal exercises progressively increase the intensity of resistance against the contraction of the abdominal muscles in the Hollow-Tank Posture.

A. Hollow Tank with Stretch

1. Lie flat on the back, knees up. Clench the hands at the shoulders, keeping them on the floor.

2. Contract the abdominal muscles and take the Hollow Tank.

3. Press up with clenched hands and down with the heels (toes up) as in the Stretching Exercise (Pages 56–57). Maintain Hollow Tank until stretch is completed.

4. Release the contraction (Hollow Tank) and inhale.

Take several breaths and repeat.

B. Hollow Tank in Spine Balance

1. Lie flat on the back and take the Hollow Tank.

2. While maintaining the Hollow Tank, lift the legs and the back a short way from the floor, keeping them rigid until a strong inner vibration is felt.

3. Return to the floor, release the contraction and inhale.

Repeat after a few normal breaths.

Suggestions for Practice

The Spine Balance should be held only as long as the contraction can be maintained. Try not to let go of the abdominal muscles.

The back and legs must be held entirely rigid, head and neck in line with the spine. Do not let the head come forward.

C. Hollow Tank with Raised Legs

1. Lie flat on the back. Raise the legs at right angles to the body and exhale.
2. Take the Hollow Tank.
3. Maintain the Hollow Tank and lower the legs to the floor.
4. Release the contraction and inhale.
Breathe normally a few times and repeat.

Suggestions for Practice

Be sure to keep the legs straight. The arms may be at the side or over the head. Keep the back flat, pressing it against the floor. The legs must be under control until they touch the floor.

D. Hollow Tank in Back-Stretching Posture

1. Sit upright, the legs extended straight in front.
2. Take the three Locks (including the Solar Plexus, or Hollow Tank) and hold, bending forward and grasping the toes. (See Back-Stretching Posture, Plate 8)
3. Release the Locks, inhale and return to sitting position.
Take several breaths and repeat.

Variation of Abdominal Churn (XLI)—*Lauliki*   Pages 120–121

A

1. Sit in cross-legged position, the hands on the knees.
2. Take the Hollow Tank with exhalation, drawing the abdomen in and under the right rib.
3. Thrust the abdomen diagonally forward to the left knee, simultaneously releasing the contraction and inhaling.
4. Contract and pull the abdomen under the left rib, exhaling.
5. Thrust the abdomen diagonally forward to the right knee, releasing the contraction and inhaling.
This constitutes one round. Repeat several rounds.
See suggestions for practice for *Abdominal Churn.*

Note. This exercise is a preparation for the *Abdominal Muscle-Isolation (Nauli),* Pages 123–124.

Part III—*Key Outline*

General Suggestions

To OBTAIN the best results in Yoga, other activities should be curtailed or if possible suspended at the beginning of the practice (especially social affairs that dissipate physical and mental energies). This should be an intensive period of work on *oneself*.

The ideal preparation is first to concentrate on cleaning out the system. This is done in two ways: through diet and internal cleansing.

The following routine is recommended:

During the first week eat mainly fruits and vegetables, preferably uncooked, some protein, but no starch or sugar. Avoid all rich foods, smoking, stimulants, and excess of any kind. Drink plenty of water, get extra sleep and rest, and as much fresh air as possible. The colon should be cleaned out daily as described on page 128.

Following this preparatory period, the colon cleansing should continue biweekly for a month or two longer. Thereafter, in order to maintain the same standard of cleanliness, it is advisable to continue flushing out the colon occasionally. Such a routine is not habit-forming, nor will it upset the regular bowel activity. On the contrary, if done in the prescribed manner, it will encourage normal evacuation and a more thorough elimination.

Suggestions for Practicing the Exercises

1. First memorize the sequence.
2. Practice until the routine can be done within the time limits indicated.
3. Increase the time and number of repetitions according to individual capacity.

In beginning the work, the routines should not be practiced too rigidly as to time. Intelligent adaptation to personal needs should always be followed. Some of the Postures and exercises may be more difficult for certain people than for others, and therefore more time and effort should be devoted to those particular practices.

Regularity is of utmost importance. Five or ten minutes of daily work will bring better results than occasional hours of desultory exercise. But a half hour is the minimum time requirement for continuous improvement.

The morning routine should be done in the sequence listed, as this is designed to progessively arouse and increase all the physical functions, until at the end of the working period the circulation and every part of the body is stimulated and toned up, ready for the day's activities.

For evening practice the routine may be done in reverse order, thus gradually diminishing activity until a deep relaxation is attained in preparation for sleep. The Rhythmic Breathing is especially conducive to sleep, and may be added at the finish of the evening exercises, or just before retiring.

Practice very slowly and intensely. Fewer times with greater concentration will prove more effective than many repetitions in hurried sequence.

A suggested routine will be found on page 168. As proficiency is gained and greater ease established, other Postures and exercises may be added, thus making the work varied and always new and interesting.

KEY OUTLINE

This outline gives a brief summary of each of the exercises, and is intended as a reference chart for daily practice. It should be used only after the detailed instructions in Part II have been studied and thoroughly understood.

Relaxation Posture   Page 55
1. Lie flat on floor. Relax completely.
2. Draw several slow, deep breaths.
3. Tense the entire body, then "let go" in every part.
4. Feel the body extremely heavy, then light as air.

Preparatory Exercises

Stretches   Page 56
1. Lie flat on floor and stretch all over.
2. Stretch right arm up, right leg down. Then opposite side.
3. Diagonal stretch: left arm, right leg; right arm, left leg.
4. Stretch up with both arms, down with both heels.

Spine Rock   Page 58
1. Sit cross-legged. Bend forward, grasping feet.
2. Rock back on spine and onto shoulders, legs over head.
3. Rock forward again to sitting position.
A. Spine Rock without holding feet.
B. Spine Rock keeping legs straight.
C. Spine Rock rising to feet.

Leg Folding   Page 59
1. Lie on back, bend knee, and fold leg back against hip.
2. Straighten leg, then bend in other direction, and place foot on opposite groin.
3. Bend knee upward against chest.
4. Straighten leg at right angles to body and pull back.
A1. Sit erect, both legs extended. Then fold back as in last exercise.
2. Same as No. 2 in last exercise.
3. Grasp heel and extend leg outward until knee is straight.
4. Lower leg slowly to floor, still holding heel.
B. Same sequence, grasping toe instead of heel.

Knee Limbering   Page 60
1. Kneel and sit on heels
2. Lift hips and sit to *right* of heels.

3. Return to first position.
4. Lift hips and sit to *left* of heels.
5. Return to first position.

Variation

A1. Sit as above, then push *feet* out to *right* side of hips.
2. Extend legs forward.
3. Bend knees and bring feet to *left* side of hips.
4. Return to kneeling position, completing square.

THE LOCKS

A. Solar-Plexus Lock   Page 61
1. Contract abdomen at pit of stomach.
2. Tense and hold.

B. Chin Lock (or Throat Lock)   Page 62
1. Press chin forcibly into notch at base of throat.
2. Tense and hold.

C. Rectal Lock   Page 62
1. Pull up and contract rectal muscles.

D. Aswini-Mudra
1. Take Rectal Lock in knee-chest position.
2. Pull in and up and force down and out alternately.

POSTURES

I. Half Posture (or Hero Posture)—*Virāsana*   Page 63
   Plate 1
1. Sit erect, fold left leg along left hip.
2. Place right foot in left groin.
3. Hold and take three Locks.
4. Repeat, reversing position of legs.

Variation   Page 132

1. Sit in Half Posture.
2. Grasp right heel with right hand, extend leg forward and up.
3. Lower leg to floor in slow extension.
4. Repeat with left leg.

II. "V" Posture—*Samkatāsana*   Page 64   Plates 2, 3
  1. Sit with legs extended.
  2. Bend left leg and place on right thigh.
  3. Cross right leg under left thigh. Press hands against knees.
  4. Hold and take three Locks.

Variations   Page 132

("V" Twist, or High Corkscrew turn)
  A1. From "V" Posture rise to left knee.
   2. Half pivot right to standing position.
   3. Continue pivoting and return to left knee.
   4. Return to "V" posture, left knee under.
(Low Corkscrew turn)
  B. Same sequence without rising.

III. Frog Posture—*Mandukāsana*   Page 67   Plate 4
  1. Sit on heels in squatting position.
  2. Fold arms at chest or over head.
  3. Hold posture and take three Locks.

Variations   Page 133

  A1. Take Frog Posture.
   2. Roll slowly forward to knees.
   3. Roll back to toes.
  B1. Take Frog Posture.
   2. Rise slowly, maintaining position on toes.
   3. While standing, rock from toes to heels and back again.
   4. Slowly bend knees and return to Frog Posture.

IV. Crossed Posture—*Bhadrāsana*   Page 68   Plate 5
  1. Kneel and sit back on crossed feet.
  2. Fold arms across the back and grasp toes.
  3. Take Chin Lock and hold posture.
  4. Repeat, reversing position of hands and feet.

V. Spine-Twist Posture—*Ardya-Matsyendrāsana*   Page 69
    Plates 6, 7
  1. Sit with legs extended.
  2. Place left foot to side of right thigh, knee close to chest.
  3. Bend right knee and bring leg close to left thigh.

4. Twist waist and hook right shoulder over left knee.
5. Repeat, reversing position.

Variation   Page 134

Same posture, but with one leg extended instead of bent back (easier for beginners).

VI. Back-stretching Posture—*Pacshimottanāsana*   Page 71
Plates 8, 9

1. Sit with legs extended.
2. Bend forward and grasp toes.
3. Bring elbows to floor and head to knees.
4. Hold posture and take three Locks.

Variations   Page 134

A1. Sit with legs extended.
   2. Stretch arms over head, swing down and touch toes.
   3. Return to sitting position, elbows back, chest open.
   4. Repeat several times.

B1. Same exercise. Exhale on forward swing.
   2. Inhale on bending elbows, as body is straightened.
   3. Hold inhalation and stretch arms over head.
   4. Return to first position (exhaling) and repeat.

(Plate 11)
C1. Sit with legs extended.
   2. Bend forward and grasp toes.
   3. Pull heels off floor.
   4. Hold and take three Locks.

(Plate 10)
D1. Stand erect, feet together.
   2. Bend forward, clasping hands behind ankles.
   3. Touch head to knees.
   4. Hold and take three Locks.

E1. Sit with legs extended.
   2. Bend forward and grasp toes.
   3. Raise legs as far off floor as possible.
   4. Balance on spine and hold.

VII. Locked Posture—*Maha-Mudra*   Page 74   Plate 11
1. Sit with legs extended.
2. Place heel of left foot against perineum.
3. Bend forward and grasp toe of right foot.
4. Take three Locks with breath suspended.
5. Repeat with opposite leg extended.

VIII. Pelvic Posture—*Vajrāsana*   Page 75   Plate 12
1. Kneel and sit between the thighs.
2. Fold legs back against the hips.
3. Hold posture and take three Locks.

Variations   Page 135

A1. Take Pelvic Posture, knees close together.
  2. Turn insteps down, arch on floor.
  3. Open heels so that arches of feet form basket for hips to
sit in.

B1. From Pelvic Posture rise slowly to knees.
  2. Return to Pelvic Posture without bending at waist.
  3. Repeat several times.

C1. Same as B, but leaning backward from hips.
  2. Repeat several times.

(Plate 13)

D1. Take Pelvic Posture, grasp insteps and rise to knees.
  2. Arch spine and bend head back between shoulders.
  3. Return to Pelvic Posture.

(Plate 14)

E1. From Pelvic Posture lean back until head touches floor.
  2. Return to knees, keeping back arched.

(The Duck Waddle)

F1. From Pelvic Posture shift weight to left leg.
  2. Bring right knee to chest, foot on floor.
  3. Bring left knee to chest, left foot on floor. (Frog Posture II)
  4. Return to Pelvic Posture in reverse order.

G1. Take Pelvic Posture and place hands on floor.
  2. With slight spring lift legs to Frog Posture.
  3. With another spring return to Pelvic Posture.

H1. From Pelvic Posture jump to Frog Posture as above.
  2. Keeping weight on hands, kick straight back.
  3. With slight spring lift legs and return to Frog Posture.
  4. From Frog Posture return to Pelvic Posture as above.

IX. Supine-Pelvic Posture—*Supta-Vajrāsana*   Page 78
   Plate 15
   1. Take Pelvic Posture.
   2. Lean back and lie flat on floor.
   3. Hold posture and take three Locks.

Variations   Page 137

A1. Take Supine-Pelvic Posture, raise knees, feet on floor.
  2. Grasp ankles, arch back and raise hips and shoulders from floor.
  3. Still holding ankles raise and lower trunk several times.

The Crab (Plate 17)
B1. Take Supine-Pelvic Posture and raise knees as above.
  2. Place hands palms down at side of shoulders. (Plate 16)
  3. Push up, raising shoulders, back and hips, until elbows are straight, head dropping back between shoulders. (Plate 17)
  4. Lower body by bending elbows and knees, returning to Supine-Pelvic Posture.

(Plate 18)
C1. Take Crab Posture and extend one leg straight up or bent.
  2. Repeat with opposite leg extended.

D1. Stand with feet 12 inches apart, arms over head.
  2. Bend backward until hands touch floor.
  3. Return to upright position.

X. Cobra Posture—*Bhujangāsana*   Page 80   Plate 19
   1. Lie face downward.
   2. Place hands on floor at shoulder level, palms down.
   3. Press body up from hips, arching backward.
   4. Hold and take three Locks.

Variations   Page 139

A1. Take Cobra Posture.
  2. Swing upper body in large circle to right and backward.

3. Continue to left, then forward, chest touching floor.

4. Repeat, circling to left.

B1. Take Cobra Posture.

2. Walk around on hands to right side of body.

3. Repeat to the left.

C1. Take Cobra Posture.

2. Press back into kneeling posture, chest to floor.

3. Sit on feet, shoulders to knees, head touching floor.

4. Return to Cobra Posture, keeping chest to floor throughout.

XI. Locust Posture—*Salabhāsana*   Page 82   Plate 20

1. Lie face downward, arms at sides, forehead and chest on floor.

2. Press palms down, arch back and lift legs up from hips.

3. Hold.

Variations   Page 139

A1. Lie face downward, hands clasped behind head.

2. Press legs up from hips, head up against pressure of hands.

3. Hold.

B1. Take Locust Posture, arms stretched diagonally up and forward.

2. Roll over on hips to Spine-Balance Posture. (XIII)

3. Roll back to first position.

4. Repeat, opposite direction.

XII. Bow Posture—*Dhanurāsana*   Page 83   Plate 21

1. Lie face downward.

2. Grasp toes, arching back.

3. Hold.

Variations   Page 140

A1. Take Bow Posture.

2. Rock back and forth on abdomen.

B1. Lie face downward.

2. Cross legs at ankles, grasp toes and arch backward.

3. Hold, or rock back and forth as in A.

XIII. Spine-Balance Posture—*Vajroli Mudra*   Page 84
Plate 22

1. Sit with legs extended, hands on floor at hips.

2. Lift legs high, press hands down, and balance on end of spine.
3. Hold.

Variations   Page 140

(Plate 23)
A1. Lie flat on back.
  2. Raise body and legs, balancing on end of spine.
  3. Hold.

(Low Spine Balance)
B1. Take posture as above. (A2)
  2. Tuck knees to chest in jackknife position.
  3. Return to first position. Repeat several times.

C1. Take posture as in A2. (Low Spine Balance)
  2. Open and close legs like scissors.

D1. Take posture as in A2. (Low Spine Balance)
  2. Pedal with legs.

E1. Take posture as in A2. (Low Spine Balance)
  2. Roll to right hip and bring knees up in jackknife position.
  3. Extend legs and roll to opposite hip and jackknife.
  4. Return to first position and repeat in opposite direction.

INVERTED POSTURES

XIV. Shoulder Stand—*Sarvangāsana*   Page 85
   Plate 24
1. Lie flat on back.
2. Slowly raise legs, then hips, then shoulders.
3. Place hands at small of back and press up.
4. Stretch up with legs and hold.

Variations   Page 141

A1. Take Shoulder Stand, keeping hands on floor.
  2. Hold.

B1. Take Shoulder Stand, with arms over head.
  2. Hold.

C1. Take Shoulder Stand.
  2. Bend knees in jackknife position to right shoulder.

3. Straighten knees and bend to left shoulder.
4. Return to first position.
D1. Take Shoulder Stand.
  2. Tense leg muscles, then relax and shake.
E1. Take Shoulder Stand.
  2. Open and close legs like scissors.
F1. Take Shoulder Stand.
  2. Pedal as if riding a bicycle.

XV. Plough Posture—_Halāsana_   Page 87   Plate 25
  1. Lie flat on floor.
  2. Raise legs as in Shoulder Stand.
  3. Bring legs over head until toes touch the floor.
  4. Hold.

Variations   Page 142

A1. Take Plough Posture.
  2. Place arms over head, clasping elbows.
  3. Push toes further over head, making furrows.
  4. Continue "ploughing."
(Plate 26)
B1. Take Plough Posture.
  2. Bend knees and bring to shoulders.
  3. Hold.
C1. Take Shoulder Stand.
  2. Bring legs alternately over head, touching floor.
D1. Take Shoulder Stand.
  2. Lower legs very slowly to Plough Posture.
  3. Return slowly to Shoulder Stand.
E1. Take Shoulder Stand.
  2. Swing right leg over left shoulder, touching floor.
  3. Swing left leg over right shoulder, touching floor.
F1. Take Shoulder Stand.
  2. Swing both legs over right shoulder, touching floor.
  3. Repeat, with legs over left shoulder.
G1. Take Plough Posture.
  2. Circle with legs, touching floor over head, sides and front.
  3. Repeat in opposite direction.

XVI. Head Stand—*Sirshāsana*   Page 89   Plates 27, 28, 29
Triangle
1. Kneel, head touching floor, hands overlapping around head.
2. Straighten legs and walk up till knees touch chest.
3. Tuck knees up and push off floor with toes, arching back.
4. Straighten legs upwards slowly.
5. Return slowly to first position.

Tripod   (Plate 30)
1. Kneel, head on floor, hands placed in front of knees.
2. Straighten legs and walk up, knees to chest.
3. Place knees on elbows, feet off floor.
4. Lift legs slowly to straight position.
5. Return slowly to first position.

Variations   Page 143

Swastika   (Plate 30)
A1. Stand, lunge forward on right leg, dropping to left knee.
  2. Rock forward to right knee.
  3. Place head and arms in triangle position.
  4. Swing left leg over head, knee bent.
  5. Lift right leg over head, knee bent.

Willow Tree
B1. Take Triangle Head Stand.
  2. Open the legs and bend knees over the head.

Jackknife
C1. Take Willow-Tree Head Stand.
  2. Tuck knees to chest, reversing arch of spine.
  3. Return to Willow-Tree position.

Splits in Head Stand
D1. Take Triangle Head Stand.
  2. Open and close legs. (Front Split)
  3. Open and close legs to the side. (Side Split)
  4. Bicycle with legs, remaining in Head Stand.

Pull-up Head Stand
E1. Lie face downward, arms in Triangle position.
  2. Pull up into Head Stand, keeping legs straight.
  3. Return slowly to first position.

MEDITATION POSTURES

XVII. Perfect Posture—*Siddhāsana*   Page 95   Plate 32
 1. Sit with legs outstretched.
 2. Place right heel at crotch of left leg.
 3. Place left heel over right heel.
 4. Hold.

Variations   Page 144

A1. From Perfect Posture rise to knees, arms folded over head.
  2. Open legs backward and sit in Pelvic Posture.
  3. Return, rising to knees, feet folded under.
  4. Sit back in Perfect Posture.

(Plate 33)
B1. Bring soles of feet together, knees flat on floor.
  2. Place hands together at chest.

XVIII. Hidden Posture—*Guptāsana*   Page 96   Plate 34
 1. Sit with legs outstretched.
 2. Place right tocs in left knee joint.
 3. Bring left foot under, toes in bend of right knee.
 4. Hold.

XIX. Lotus Posture—*Padmāsana*   Page 97   Plate 35
 1. Sit with legs outstretched.
 2. Place right foot on top of left thigh at groin.
 3. Place left foot on top of right thigh at groin.
 4. Hold.

ADVANCED POSTURES

XX. Completed Lotus Posture—*Baddha Padmāsana*   Page 98
    Plate 36
 1. Take Lotus Posture.
 2. Cross left arm behind back and grasp left toe.
 3. Cross right arm behind back and grasp right toe.
 4. Hold.

XXI. Lotus Head Stand—*Sirshāsana Padmāsana*   Page 100
   Plates 37, 38, 39
   1. Take Lotus Posture.
   2. Rock forward on to knees.
   3. Place head and hands in Tripod position.
   4. Slide knees up onto elbows.
   5. Lift folded legs into Head Stand position.

XXII. Symbolical Posture—*Yoga Mudra*   Page 102
   Plate 40
   1. Take Lotus Posture.
   2. Bend forward and touch head to floor.
   3. Stretch arms forward and touch hands to floor, or clasp hands
at back and touch head to floor.
   4. Hold.

XXIII. Fish Posture—*Matsyāsana*   Page 104   Plate 41
   1. Take Lotus Posture.
   2. Lie back flat on floor, hands grasping toes.
   3. Arch neck and shoulders, rolling onto top of head.
   4. Hold.

XXIV. Cock Posture—*Kukkutāsana*   Page 105   Plate 42
   1. Take Lotus Posture.
   2. Place hands beside hips and press up off floor.
   3. Hold, resting only on hands.

XXV. Peacock Posture—*Mayurāsana*   Page 106   Plate 43
   1. Take Lotus Posture.
   2. Place hands in front and roll up to knees.
   3. Hook elbows in pelvic hollows above hip bones.
   4. Press up, balancing on hands and hold.

XXVI. Tree, or Stork Posture—*Vriksāsana*   Page 107
   Plate 44
   1. Stand Erect.
   2. Place right foot in opposite groin.
   3. Bring arms above head, palms together.
   4. Balance and hold. (Repeat with opposite leg)

BREATHING PRACTICES

XXVII. Deep-Cleansing Breath   Page 109
1. Sit in any Meditation Posture, or cross-legged.
2. Exhale forcibly through mouth, bringing arms and head to floor.
3. Inhale through nose, returning to sitting posture, arms circling to back, palms pressed to floor.
4. Retain breath a few seconds, then repeat.

XXVIII. Alternate, or Nasal-Cleansing Breath—*Vama-Krama*
     Page 109
1. Close right nostril with right thumb, inhaling through left nostril.
2. Close left nostril with fingers and retain breath a few seconds with both nostrils closed.
3. Remove right thumb from right nostril and exhale, keeping left nostril closed.
4. Inhale forcibly through right nostril.
5. Close right nostril with right thumb and retain breath a few seconds with both nostrils closed.
6. Remove fingers from left nostril and exhale, keeping right nostril closed.

XXIX. Rhythmic Breath   Page 110
1. Inhale through nose (4 counts).
2. Retain breath and take three Locks (16 counts).
3. Release Locks and exhale through nose (8 counts).

XXX. Rhythmic Alternate Breath   Page 111
1. Inhale through left nostril (4 counts).
2. Retain breath, both nostrils closed (16 counts).
3. Exhale through right nostril (left closed—8 counts).
4. Inhale through right nostril (left closed—4 counts).
5. Retain breath, both nostrils closed (16 counts).
6. Exhale through left nostril (right closed—8 counts).

XXXI. Bellows Breath—*Bhastrika*   Page 111
1. Expel breath through nostrils, contracting abdomen.
2. Release contraction, automatically taking in air.

3. Follow immediately with another forcible expulsion.

4. Repeat a number of times in immediate succession.

5. Inhale to capacity, swallow and take three Locks. Hold the breath.

6. Exhale very slowly, releasing pressure gradually.

XXXII. Sighing Breath—*Ujjayi*　　Page 113

1. Draw breath forcibly through nose, making a sighing sound.

2. Exhale forcibly and evenly, continuing same sound.

XXXIII. Hissing, or Swan Breath—*Sitali,* or *Hamsa*　　Page 113

1. Inhale forcibly through nose.

2. With lips pressed against teeth expel with hissing sound.

XXXIV. Droning Breath—*Brahmari*　　Page 113

1. Inhale forcibly through nose.

2. With slightly parted lips expel wth low humming sound.

A1. Inhale forcibly through nose.

2. Place fingers over ears, eyelids, nostrils, upper and lower lips.

3. Exhale with low humming sound, as above.

XXXV. Stretching Breath　　Page 114　　Plate 45

1. Take kneeling posture, head and shoulders touching floor.

2. Inhale, rising to knees, arms over head stretching upward.

3. Retain breath, clasp left wrist with right hand and pull over to right side.

4. Still retaining breath repeat stretch to left side.

5. Still retaining breath return to central position, unclasp hands and make big circle bringing hands together at back.

6. Slowly exhale and return to kneeling position in reverse order.

ABDOMINAL EXERCISES

XXXVI. Hollow Tank—*Tadagi-Mudra*　　Page 116　　Plate 46

1. Lie flat on back, knees up, feet on floor.

2. Exhale vigorously through mouth.

3. With breath out pull abdomen in and up.

4. Hold, then release contraction and inhale.

XXXVII. Pelvic Hollow Tank—*Vajroli-Mudra*   Page 118
   Plate 22
   1. Lie flat on floor, arms at side.
   2. Exhale and take Hollow Tank.
   3. Raise trunk and legs into jackknife position, hands pressing down.
   4. Hold, then release tension and inhale, returning to first position.

XXXVIII. Abdominal Lift   Page 118   Plate 47
   1. Lie on back, knees bent, weight on elbows.
   2. Take Hollow Tank, simultaneously exhaling.
   3. Release and expand with inhalation.

XXXIX. Hammock Swing   Page 119
   1. Lie flat on back.
   2. Exhale, simultaneously contracting and lifting abdominal muscles.
   3. Inhale, simultaneously releasing contraction and pushing abdomen right.
   4. Exhale and again contract.
   5. Inhale and push abdomen left.

XL. Cat Hump   Page 119   Plate 48
   1. Take position on hands and knees.
   2. Exhale, simultaneously contracting and lifting abdominal muscles, arching back up like a cat.
   3. Inhale, simultaneously releasing contraction and pushing abdomen down, reversing arch in back. Repeat a number of times.
   A. Same exercise with Hammock Swing.

XLI. Abdominal Churn—*Lauliki*   Page 120
   1. Sit cross-legged, hands on knees.
   2. Exhale, simultaneously contracting and lifting abdominal muscles.
   3. Rotate abdominal muscles in circular motion, first to right, then to left.

XLII. Power Whip—*Uddiyhana*   Page 121   Plate 49
   1. Stand with legs apart, knees bent, hands pressing against thighs.

2. Exhale vigorously, taking Hollow Tank (XXXVI)

3. Holding breath out, whip abdomen in and immediately release.

4. Repeat a number of times before again inhaling.

Variation

A. Same exercise sitting in cross-legged position.

XLIII. Abdominal Muscle Isolation—*Nauli*   Page 123
    Plate 50

1. Stand with legs apart, knees bent, hands pressing against thighs.

2. Take Hollow Tank with vigorous exhalation.

3. With breath out, press out first right abdominal muscle then left.

4. Repeat a number of times before again inhaling.

CLEANSING PRACTICES

XLIV. Nasal Cleansing—*Sit Krama* or *Matangini-Mudra—*
    "Elephant" *Mudra*   Page 125

1. Fill mouth full of water.

2. Bend head well forward over basin.

3. Expel water through nose.

XLV. Tongue Cleansing—*Jihva-Sodhana* or *Tongue Dhauti*
    Page 125

1. Extend tongue out as far forward as possible.

2. Massage vigorously with fingers at base of tongue.

Tongue Stretching

A1. Grasp tongue with towel or piece of cloth.

  2. Stretch and pull forward.

XLVI. Stomach Cleansing—*Vamana-Dhauti*   Page 126

1. Drink 6 to 8 glasses luke-warm water.

2. Do Power-Whip exercise (XLII).

3. Open throat and press tongue down.

4. Expel as forcibly as possible.

XLVII. Colon Cleansing—*Basti*   Page 128

1. Take low enema, expelling immediately.

2. While in knee-chest position take two-quart enema.

3. Retain water and do as many of the abdominal exercises as possible.

4. Eliminate and continue abdominal exercises until all water is expelled.

XLVIII. Air Cleansing—*Vatasara-Dhauti*   Page 130

Crow Bill Mudra

A1. Contract mouth, lips protruding, and suck in air.

2. When mouth is full of air, open throat and swallow forcibly.

3. Repeat several times until stomach is filled with air.

4. Do abdominal exercises, gradually forcing air out through rectum.

B1. Open throat wide, at same time contracting abdominal muscles in Hollow Tank.

2. Vacuum thus created will suck air directly into stomach without swallowing.

Plavini-Mudra   Page 130

C1. Fill the stomach with air, as above.

2. Take Fish Posture, with back flat, arms locked above head.

Suggested Routine

		PAGE		
1.	Relaxation Posture	55	1	min.
2.	Stretches	56	1½	min.
3.	Nasal-Cleansing Breath (XXVIII)	109 (4 times)	1½	min.
4.	Deep Cleansing Breath (XXVII)	109 (6 times, hold)	2	min.
5.	Spine Rock	58 (6 times)	½	min.
6.	Leg Folding	59 (twice each side)	2	min.
7.	Variations (A or B)	60 (6 times)	2	min.
8.	Frog Posture (A & B) (III)	133 (4 times each)	1½	min.
9.	Pelvic Posture (VIII)	75 (hold)		
	Pelvic Posture (Var. B)	135 (4 times)	1½	min.
10.	Relaxation Posture	55	1	min.
11.	Back-Stretching Post. (A & B) (VI)	134 (4 times each)	2	min.
12.	Cobra Posture (X)	80 (hold)		
	Cobra Posture (Var. A)	139 (4 times each dir.)	1½	min.
13.	Bow Posture (XII)	83 (hold)	1	min.
14.	Spine-Balance Posture (A) (XIII)	140 (4 times)	1	min.*
15.	Shoulder Stand (XIV)	85 (hold)		*
	Shoulder Stand (Var. D)	141 (4 times)	1½	min.
16.	Plough Posture (XV)	87 (4 times)	1½	min.
17.	Deep Cleansing Breath (XXVII)	109 (6 times, hold)	2	min.
18.	Hollow Tank (XXXVI)	116 (4 times, hold)	1½	min.
19.	Abdominal Lift (XXXVIII)	118 (15 times)	1	min.
20.	Cat Hump (XL)	119 (15 times)	1	min.
21.	Head Stand (1 & 2 only) (XVI)	89 (2 times, hold)	1½	min.*
22.	Bellows Breath (XXXI)	111 (20 times, hold)	1½	min.*
23.	Relaxation Posture	55	1	min.

33 min.

* Gradually increase holding time.

Books on Yoga

Aurobindo, Sri, *The Synthesis of Yoga.*
Avalon, Arthur, *Principles of Tantra.*
Idem, Serpent Power.
Behanon, K. T. *Yoga; a Scientific Evaluation,* New York, The Macmillan Co.
Bernard, Theos, *Hatha Yoga,* New York, Columbia University Press.
Idem, Heaven Lies Within Us, New York, Charles Scribner's Sons.
Idem, Hindu Philosophy, New York, Philosophical Library, Inc.
Evans-Wentz, *Tibetan Book of the Dead,* New York, Oxford University Press, Inc.
Idem, Tibetan Yoga & Secret Doctrines, New York, Oxford University Press, Inc.
Idem, Tibetan Book of the Great Liberation, New York, Oxford University Press, Inc.
Goddard, Dwight, *The Buddhist Bible.*
Kuvalayananda, *Asanas.*
Idem, Pranayama.
Rele, V. G., *The Mysterious Kundalini.*
Idem, Yogic Asanas.
Vithaldas, *The Yoga System of Health,* London, Faber & Faber, Ltd.
Vivekananda, *Collected Works.*
Wilhelm, R., *The Secret of the Golden Flower,* New York, Harcourt, Brace & Co.
Wood, Ernest, *A Yoga Dictionary,* New York, Philosophical Library.
Idem, Great Systems of Yoga, New York, Philosophical Library.
Idem, Practical Yoga, Ancient and Modern, New York, E. P. Dutton.
Woodroffe, Sir John, *Shakti, Shakta.*
Idem, The Garland of Letters.
Woods, J. H., *The Yoga System of Patanjali,* Cambridge, Mass., Harvard University Press.
Yesudian & Heatch, *Yoga and Health,* New York, Harper & Brothers.

The Baghavad Gita, Idem.

The Crest Jewel of Wisdom.
Patanjali Aphorisms, Translated by Sw. Prabhavananda & Isherwood.

Related (or Supplementary) Reading

Arnold, Sir Edwin, *Light of Asia.*
Idem, Song Celestial
Benoit, Hubert, *The Supreme Doctrine,* New York, Pantheon Books, Inc.
Fromm, Eric, *Man for Himself,* New York, Rinehart & Co.
Gervis, Pearce, *Naked They Pray.*
Heard, Gerald, *Pain, Sex, and Time,* New York, Harper & Brothers.
Idem, The Eternal Gospel, New York, Harper & Brothers.
Huxley, Aldous, *The Perennial Philosophy,* New York, Harper & Brothers.
Isherwood, editor, *Vedanta for the Western World,* Hollywood, Calif., Marcel Rodd Co.
Jung, C. G., *Modern Man in Search of a Soul.*
Idem, Religion of the East & West.
Krishnamurti, J., *The First and Last Freedom,* New York, Harper & Brothers.
Nicoll, Maurice, *Living Time,* Vincent & Stuart.
Ouspensky, P. D., *A New Model of the Universe.*
Powys, John Cowper, *The Meaning of Culture,* New York, W. W. Norton & Co., Inc.
Idem, The Philosophy of Solitude, New York, Simon & Schuster, Inc.
Watts, Allan, *The Supreme Identity,* London, Faber & Faber, Ltd.